SUBSTANCE ABUSE AND PHYSICAL DISABILITY

Allen W. Heinemann, PhD
Editor

SOME ADVANCE REVIEWS

"Destined to become a standard text for those aspiring to facilitate change in persons with this vexing dual-disability. A wealth of clinical and research knowledge has been assembled in this text, providing a conceptual and procedural framework for effective intervention. . . . Provocative and challenging . . . I highly recommend this text to anyone working with disabled clients for whom substance abuse has emerged as a maladaptive coping strategy."

Mervin J. Langley, PhD
Director, Neurological and Addictive Behavior Services
New Medico Rehabilitation Center of Wisconsin

"A seminal contribution . . . Heinemann has artfully melded sixteen chapters into a fast yet smoothly paced presentation which is simultaneously authoritative and comprehensive. Helps fill what has until now been a significant gap in the literature. It will undoubtedly come to be recognized as a significant contribution to the rehabilitation and addiction literatures."

M. G. Eisenberg, PhD, Editor, Rehabilitation Technology
Chief, Psychology Service, VA Medical Center
Hampton, Virginia

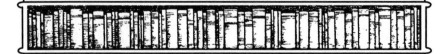

Substance Abuse
and Physical Disability

HAWORTH Addictions Treatment
F. Bruce Carruth, PhD
Senior Editor

New, Recent, and Forthcoming Titles:

Group Psychotherapy with Addicted Populations by Philip J. Flores

Shame, Guilt and Alcoholism: Treatment Issues in Clinical Practice by Ronald T. Potter-Efron

Neuro-Linguistic Programming in Alcoholism Treatment edited by Chelly M. Sterman

Cocaine Solutions: Help for Cocaine Abusers and Their Families by Jennifer Rice-Licare and Katherine Delaney-McLoughlin

Preschoolers and Substance Abuse: Strategies for Prevention and Intervention by Pedro J. Lecca and Thomas D. Watts

Addiction in Human Development: Developmental Perspectives on Addiction and Recovery by Jacqueline Wallen

Chemical Dependency and Antisocial Personality Disorder: Psychotherapy and Assessment Strategies by Gary G. Forrest

Substance Abuse and Physical Disability edited by Allen W. Heinemann

Substance Abuse and Physical Disability

Allen W. Heinemann, PhD
Editor

The Haworth Press
New York • London • Norwood (Australia)

Support for this text was provided by the National Institute on Disability and Rehabilitation Research, United States Department of Education, as part of a Field Initiated Project grant to the editor.

The Haworth Press, Inc., 10 Alice Street, Binghamton, NY 13904-1580

Library of Congress Cataloging-in-Publication Data

Substance abuse and physical disability / Allen W. Heinemann.
     p.   cm.
     Includes bibliographical references and index.
     ISBN 1-56024-289-2 (alk. paper).
     1. Physically handicapped–Substance use. 2. Substance abuse–Treatment. I. Heinemann, Allen W.
     [DNLM: 1. Alcoholism. 2. Handicapped. 3. Substance Abuse.
WM 270 S940457]
RC564.5.P48S83   1992
616.86′0087–dc20
DNLM/DLC
for Library of Congress   92–1443
                                                              CIP

CONTENTS

PART III: ASSESSMENT, TREATMENT, AND PREVENTION ISSUES

ABOUT THE EDITOR

Allen W. Heinemann, PhD, is Associate Professor of Physical Medicine and Rehabilitation at Northwestern University Medical School and Director of the Rehabilitation Services Evaluation Unit at the Rehabilitation Institute of Chicago. He is a past faculty member of the Rehabilitation Counseling and Psychology programs at the Illinois Institute of Technology. Dr. Heinemann is a member of the American Psychological Association, division of Rehabilitation Psychology, the American Congress of Rehabilitation Medicine, the American Rehabilitation Counseling Association, and the Research Society on Alcoholism. He received his PhD in Clinical Psychology, with a specialty in Rehabilitation Psychology, from the University of Kansas.

About the Contributors

Thomas Babor, PhD is a Professor in the Department of Psychiatry, University of Connecticut School of Medicine, and serves as Scientific Director of the Alcohol Research Center, Farmington, Connecticut. His current research interests include screening, diagnosis, early intervention, and treatment evaluation, as well as cultural factors related to alcohol problems. Dr. Babor received his doctoral degree in social psychology from the University of Arizona in 1971. He spent several years in postdoctoral research training in social psychiatry at Harvard Medical School, and subsequently served as head of social science research at McLean Hospital's Alcohol and Drug Abuse Research Center in Belmont, Massachusetts. In 1977, he received a research scientists development award from the National Institute on Alcohol Abuse and Alcoholism (NIAAA). During the course of this five-year program, he studied alcoholism in France, investigated determinants of alcohol self-administration, and received training in public health concepts as applied to alcohol problems. In 1982, Dr. Babor moved to the University of Connecticut School of Medicine, Farmington, Connecticut.

Michael Brandt, PhD works as a psychologist at Watertown Memorial Hospital, Watertown, Wisconsin where he is currently developing a Behavioral Medicine program. He also provides clinical outpatient services to clients with alcohol and drug related problems. He continues to conduct research in the area of alcohol and drug abuse and in the area of cardiovascular behavioral medicine. Dr. Brandt earned his doctoral degree in psychology from Illinois Institute of Technology and recently completed a postdoctoral fellowship in Behavioral Medicine at the University of Chicago.

Thomas J. Budziack, PhD is a consulting psychologist who works with clinical practice groups to develop empirically-based substance abuse treatment services. He specializes in the identification and treatment of early stage substance abuse problems and in working with difficult or resistant clients who have not complied with previous treatment efforts. Dr. Budziack earned a doctoral degree in Rehabilitation Psychology from the University of Wisconsin-Madison, and has 20 years of clinical and consulting experience in the mental health and substance abuse field. He served for two years as a Visiting Assistant Professor in the Psychology Department of the Illinois Institute of Technology, where he taught graduate courses in counseling techniques, research design, and substance abuse treatment. Dr. Budziack is a Certified Rehabilitation Counselor and a licensed psychologist in Illinois and Arizona.

Linda Cherry, BA is a social marketing and communications consultant with a particular interest in alcohol and other drug problems. Based in Hayward, California, she has consulted with the Institute on Alcohol, Drugs, and Disability since 1987 on a variety of information gathering and advocacy projects. She also consults with alcohol and drug service providers, colleges and universities, and social service agencies on promoting ideas and creating social change.

Martin Doot, MD is Vice President of Medical Services at Parkside Medical Services Corporation affiliated with the Lutheran General Health Care System. He practices addiction medicine at Parkside Lutheran Hospital and Lutheran General Hospital, Park Ridge, Illinois. He is Director of Medical Education for Parkside Lutheran Hospital and Chairman of the Review Course Committee for the American Society of Addiction Medicine. He has a teaching appointment at the University of Illinois as Assistant Professor of Family Practice. His research interest is linkages between primary care and addiction medicine.

Kenneth K. Gorman is a specialist in disability and addiction. He has consulted with rehabilitation facilities nationally regarding addiction issues. In the past he established a non-profit, Denver-based outpatient organization designed to meet the needs of the multi-disabled substance abuser. Currently he lectures to schools, rehabilitation centers and treatment facilities nationally on prevention of drinking and driving and drug abuse.

Allen W. Heinemann, PhD is an Associate Professor in the Department of Physical Medicine and Rehabilitation at Northwestern University Medical School, and Director of the Rehabilitation Services Evaluation Unit at the Rehabilitation Institute of Chicago. At the Rehabilitation Institute of Chicago he directs studies of rehabilitation outcome and cost effectiveness; consults with physicians, nurses, and allied health staff on research methodology and statistics; teaches a course in research design and methodology; and provides direct patient care as a psychologist. Prior to his RIC appointment, he was Assistant Professor of Psychology at Illinois Institute of Technology. He taught courses in research methodology and statistics, psychological measurement, medical and psychosocial aspects of disability, independent living, and a prepracticum in rehabilitation counseling at IIT. He was also a National Institute on Disability and Rehabilitation Research–Mary Switzer fellow. His graduate school preparation included an appointment at Baylor College of Medicine in Houston, Texas, where he was a psychology intern specializing in behavioral medicine and health psychology. He graduated from the clinical psychology program at the University of Kansas, specializing in rehabilitation psychology. He is a member of the American Evaluation Association, the American Congress of Rehabilitation Medicine, the American Psychological Association, the American Association for Counseling and Development, the American Rehabilitation Counseling Association, and the National Council of Rehabilitation Education; and an editorial board member for several professional journals.

Reid Hester, PhD is a Research Associate Professor at the Center for Research on Addictive Behaviors in the Department of Psychology, and Clinical Associate in the Department of Psychiatry, University of New Mexico, and Director of the Alcohol Self-Control Program at Behavior Therapy Associates in Albuquerque, New Mexico. He has been a Principal Investigator on a total of four National Insitute on Alcohol Abuse and Alcoholism (NIAAA)-funded research projects. Currently, he is a co-principal investigator on a NIAAA, multi-site cooperative alcoholism treatment outcome research project. He maintains an active clinical practice in the areas of substance abuse and behavioral medicine, and is actively involved in professional training and consultation at the national and international level. In the past, he has been a consultant to the National Institute of Alcohol Abuse and Alcoholism and the National Institute of Drug Abuse. Dr. Hester received his PhD in Clinical Psychology from Washington State University in 1979. He has been involved in research in alcohol abuse since 1974 and has published a number of literature reviews of alcoholism treatment. One of his most recent publications is *Handbook of Alcoholism Treatment Approaches: Effective Alternatives* published by Pergamon.

Lawrence K. Horberg, PhD has extensive clinical and research experience in the treatment of addiction. He is a Psychologist in Private Practice in Chicago, and an Assistant Professor in the Department of Psychiatry and Behavioral Sciences of Northwestern University Medical School, Chicago, Illinois. He has co-authored a book, *Taking Charge,* for family members of addicts. Dr. Horberg has contributed to the professional literature in this area in refereed journals and has lectured at many regional and national gatherings on his work in the treatment of addicts and their families.

Deborah Kiley, PhD is a Personal Development Manager at Andersen & Co., a leading public accounting firm. Previously she directed the Substance Abuse Prevention Program for Persons with Traumatic Head and Spinal Cord Injuries at the Rehabilitation Institute of Chicago. She earned her doctoral degree in rehabilitation psychology at Illinois Institute of Technology. She has over 13 years of experience in physical disability, substance abuse, mental health, and rehabilitation.

Sharon Schaschl, RN, BSN, CCDP is certified as a Chemical Dependency Practitioner by the Institute for Chemical Dependency Professionals of Minnesota, Inc. Her nursing background includes 16 years in rehabilitation and 11 years in chemical dependency. She has been Coordinator for the Chemical Dependency/Physical Disability Program at Abbott Northwestern Hospital/Sister Kenny Institute since 1983. She is a member of the Adjunct Faculty at Mankato State University and is a consultant/small group facilitator for the University of Minnesota Program in Human Sexuality. She is on the advisory board for Bridgeway Treatment Center and has been a member of the Advisory Committee for a State of Minnesota Grant administered by the Hazelden Foundation. She has conducted extensive training in the area of chemical dependency and physical disability throughout the United States, in Puerto Rico, and in Canada. She has co-authored an article, "Results of a Model Intervention Program for Physically Impaired Persons," which was published in *Alcohol Health and Research World* in 1989, and contributed to articles in *Rehab Management* and *Spinal Network*. Ms. Schaschl received a Bachelor of Science Degree in Nursing from the University of Connecticut.

Stephen Schlesinger, PhD has extensive clinical and research experince in the treatment of addiction. He is a Psychologist in Private Practice in Chicago and is an Assistant Professor in the Department of Psychiatry and Behavioral Sciences of Northwestern University Medical School, Chicago, Illinois. He has co-authored a book, *Taking Charge,* for family members of addicts. Dr. Schlesinger is co-author of *Stop Drinking and Start Living*, a book for problem drinkers and co-editor of a seminal family therapy book, *Cognitive-Behavioral Therapy with Families*. In addition, Dr. Schlesinger has contributed to the professional literature in this area in refereed journals and has lectured at many regional and national gatherings on their work in the treatment of addicts and their families.

Sidney Schnoll, MD, PhD is a Professor in the Departments of Medicine and Psychiatry at the Medical College of Virginia–Virginia Commonwealth University. He completed his medical degree at the New Jersey College of Medicine and his doctoral degree in Pharmacology from Thomas Jefferson University. Dr. Schnoll serves as a member of the Center for Drugs and Biologics Advisory Committee for the Food and Drug Administration and as Research Professor of Psychology at Virginia Commonwealth University. Previously, he served as chief of the Chemical Dependence Program of Northwestern Memorial Hospital in Chicago. He has published widely on treatment of cocaine abuse, the effects of perinatal substance exposure on the fetus and neonate, occupational performance and substance use, and physical disability and substance use.

Yvonne Shade-Zeldow, PhD is Director of Behavioral Medicine at the Chicago Neurosurgical Center, and Assistant Clinical Professor in the Department of Psychiatry and Behavioral Sciences at Northwestern University Medical School, Chicago, Illinois. Prior to taking her current position, Dr. Shade-Zeldow was Director of the Department of Psychology at the Rehabilitation Institute of Chicago, where she continued her clinical work in the evaluation and treatment of patients experiencing chronic and subacute pain.

Franklin Shontz, PhD is a Professor in the Department of Psychology at the University of Kansas, and consultant to the Greater Kansas City Mental Health Foundation and the Christian Psychological Services in Kansas City, Missouri. He completed his doctoral degree at Case Western Reserve University and served as director of the graduate program in rehabilitation psychology from 1960 to 1980 at the University of Kansas and as chief psychologist at the Highland View Cuyahoga County Hospital in Cleveland, Ohio, from 1954 to 1960. Recent publications include *The Psychological Aspects of Physical Illness and Disability* published by Macmillan (1975), *Cocaine Users: A Representative Case Approach* published by the Free Press (1980), as well as articles on personological approaches to understanding individuals.

Dennis Straw, CCDP is certified as a Chemical Dependency Practitioner by the Institute for Chemical Dependency Professionals of Minnesota, Inc., and has worked as a consultant in the Chemical Dependency/Physical Disability Program at Abbott Northwestern Hospital/Sister Kenny Institute since 1983. He is a member of the Adjunct Faculty at Mankato State University. He has been a member of the Advisory Committee for a State of Minnesota Grant administered by the Hazelden Foundation. He was selected as a member of a national task force on Substance Abuse and Physical Disability sponsored by the Office of Substance Abuse Prevention. He has conducted extensive training in the area of chemical dependency and physical disability throughout the United States and Canada. He has co-authored an article, "Results of a Model Intervention Program for Physically Impaired Persons," which was published in *Alcohol Health and Research World* in 1989, and contributed to an article in *Spinal Network*. He has a disability and is recovering from chemical dependency. He was an honor student at the University of Minnesota in the School of Management.

Gary M. Yarkony, MD is the Director of Spinal Cord Injury Rehabilitation and attending physician at the Rehabilitation Institute of

Chicago. He is Clinical Associate Professor in the Department of Physical Medicine and Rehabilitation at Northwestern University Medical School. He serves as Adjunct Associate at the Pritzker Institute of Medical Engineering at Illinois Institute of Technology. Dr. Yarkony completed his medical education at the State University of New York–Upstate Medical Center in Syracuse and his residency at Northwestern University Medical School.

PART I:
UNDERSTANDING THE CONTEXT, ISSUES, AND PROBLEMS OF SUBSTANCE ABUSE

Chapter 1

An Introduction to Substance Abuse and Physical Disability

Allen W. Heinemann, PhD

Alcohol and other drug problems are national in scope and pose serious consequences in the general population. Our tendency to compartmentalize human needs, however, has made it difficult to recognize and address substance abuse problems experienced by persons with physical disabilities. Recognition of alcohol and other drug abuse as problems for persons with disabilities has been highlighted by studies that document substance use as a contributing factor in up to 68% of traumatic, disabling injuries. In addition to causing disability, the inappropriate use of alcohol or other drugs by persons with disabilities may undermine learning during rehabilitation and adversely affect rehabilitation outcomes, including general health, functional ability, attainment of vocational and educational goals, and maintenance of independent living. Clearly, alcohol and other drug problems pose significant risks to persons with disabilities.

Alcohol and other drug abuse is important to consider for several reasons. It may be a sign of poor psychosocial adjustment for persons with physical disabilities who are minimally involved in educational or vocational goals. For persons with a pre-disability history of substance abuse, it may increase the risk of post-disability substance abuse. Rehabilitation, as a process of learning to do familiar tasks in new ways, can be impaired if a person is under the influence of alcohol or other drugs. The importance of striving toward other life goals may be diminished if alcohol or other drug seeking and using becomes a primary motive. Persons with disabilities may seek drugs for the same reasons able-bodied persons do: to reduce anxiety and pain, to enhance sleep, to reduce feelings of isolation and loneliness, and to enhance a feeling of sociability and self-worth. They may have special reasons as well, such as minimizing spasticity and numbing a sense of disenfranchisement and exclusion from society.

Rehabilitation professionals may feel unqualified to address substance abuse issues, just as chemical dependence professionals feel unqualified to deal with disability issues. In part, this reflects the increased specialization within health care, even though members of the same disciplines (e.g., physicians, nurses, psychologists, social workers, vocational counselors, occupational therapists) work in both kinds of settings. This text attempts to enhance the exchange of specialized and pioneering knowledge across these fields. This requires an appreciation of clients as whole persons who experience needs in several areas simultaneously as a result of addiction, disability, and the stigma associated with these conditions.

This text is designed to provide readers with information necessary to understand the context of substance abuse in the lives of persons with disabilities, to identify chemical dependence problems, and to implement effective treatment strategies. The primary audience for this book is rehabilitation professionals: physicians, nurses, psychologists, vocational rehabilitation counselors, and allied health therapists. The text was written to serve as a single source that applies current information about substance abuse and addictions to persons with physical disabilities. A secondary audience is chemical dependence professionals; the text considers their needs for information regarding physical and cognitive disabilities.

It is easy to overlook the diversity among persons with disabilities. The kinds of characteristics that distinguish able-bodied persons, such as gender, age, race, ethnic background, education, and parental alcohol abuse, also distinguish persons with disabilities. In addition, the way in which disability is acquired (congenital vs. acquired) and the function which is limited (sensory, mobility, cognition, or affect) create specific subcultures and distinctive characteristics among persons with disabilities. Thus, the way in which substance abuse-related issues become manifest can vary greatly among persons with disabilities even as the similar risk factors they share with able-bodied persons are striking. This fact of common and unique ways in which persons with disabilities are vulnerable to substance abuse must be recognized in the organization and delivery of chemical dependence services.

The objective of this text is to present information which provides a context for understanding substance abuse issues. The material is organized into 16 chapters in four sections. The first section, titled "Understanding the Context, Issues and Problems of Substance Abuse," is comprised of three chapters including this introduction. Kenny Gorman's chapter, titled "Addicted and Disabled: One Man's Journey from Helplessness to Hope," provides an autobiographical account of chemical dependence and conveys an example of how disability and chemical dependence can be related. He reports experiencing an arduous and lengthy struggle before successfully engaging in treatment, and the ways in which rehabilitation professionals can inadvertently foster chemical dependence.

Franklin Shontz' chapter, "A Personological Integration of Chemical Dependence and Physical Disability," describes an approach to understanding whole persons with complex aspects, and provides a context within which physical disability and chemical dependence issues can be integrated. His application of personology as a way of understanding human beings as whole persons is particularly valuable in a professional arena in which seemingly disparate aspects of a person, such as disability and chemical dependence, are usually examined as part processes. He uses the case of an individual with a physical disability who abused substances to illustrate the value of understanding the life context and relatedness of different aspects of a person in acquiring a more complete view of the person. In turn, this fuller view can help professionals deal with problems such as substance abuse with a greater appreciation of their client.

In the second section, titled "Understanding the Causes, Types, and Prevalence of Substance Abuse," are five chapters dealing with nosology, typologies, and prevalence of substance use. In "Substance Use Disorders and Persons with Physical Disabilities: Nature, Diagnosis, and Clinical Subtypes," Thomas Babor presents a model of substance use disorders, describes systems of classifying substance use phenomena, and describes subtypes of alcoholism. He concludes by applying these concepts to persons with physical disabilities and highlights implications for the diagnosis, early identification, and treatment matching of persons with disabilities.

In "Prevalence and Consequences of Alcohol and Other Drug Problems Following Spinal Cord Injury," Allen Heinemann describes a series of studies that examined the prevalence of alcohol and other drug use, including prescription medications, rates of treatment for substance use, and the effects of alcohol and other drug use on the rehabilitation process and outcomes. He concludes by describing the training needs of rehabilitation professionals. Next, Sidney Schnoll describes in "Prescription Medication in Rehabilitation" several categories of prescription medications and their abuse potential, a strategy for assessing addiction, and rules for prescribing narcotic analgesics and sedative-hypnotics. He describes how persons with disabilities can achieve benefit from narcotic analgesics and sedative-hypnotics even when they have a history of substance abuse.

Gary Yarkony describes in "Medical Complications in Rehabilitation" several types of impairments resulting from trauma, frequent medical complications associated with these impairments, and the psychosocial consequences of these conditions. He provides a context for chemical dependence professionals and others who are not familiar with physical medicine and rehabilitation to understand the medical and psychosocial aspects of traumatic disability, and ways in which people with disabilities can be vulnerable to substance abuse. The last chapter in this section, "Pain Management in Rehabilitation" by Yvonne Shade-Zeldow, provides an overview of an important topic in rehabilitation: chronic pain. She defines the ways in which chronic pain eludes understanding, describes commonly used approaches in chronic pain management, operant conditioning and cognitive-behavioral techniques, and considers issues in medication management for persons experiencing chronic pain.

The third section, titled "Assessment, Treatment, and Prevention Issues," includes seven contributions. Thomas Budziack's chapter, "Substance Abuse Assessment and Treatment: Where We Are, Where We Are Going, and How It Will Affect Services to Persons with Substance Abuse Problems," describes the field of substance abuse treatment as undergoing an uneasy transition. Written primarily for rehabilitation professionals, he describes in this chapter competing conceptual models of substance abuse and dependence, and their treatment applications. The beliefs and assumptions underlying treatment approaches are analyzed, and research evidence regarding treatment effectiveness is reviewed.

Martin Doot, in "Clinical Features of Traditional Chemical Dependence Treatment Programs in the United States," describes the history of the Minnesota Model of chemical dependence treatment, and the close affiliation with Alcoholics Anonymous. The philosophy of the model, elements and structure of the Minnesota Model, procedures and guidelines for assessment, staff roles of chemical dependence treatment professionals, and issues faced by patients with both physical disabilities and chemical dependence are addressed.

In "Matching Clients to Alcohol Treatments: What Little We Know and How Very Far We Have To Go," Reid Hester describes the results of an extensive literature review on alcohol treatment outcomes, presents a hypothetical model of how client characteristics may be matched with treatment program features, emphasizes the importance of assessing client motivation to change drinking patterns, describes a six-stage model of how people may change their alcohol use, and discusses how clients can be matched with treatment programs for maximum benefit. Finally, he applies this discussion to persons with cognitive and physical disabilities.

Sharon Schaschl and Dennis Straw draw on their experience in providing substance abuse services to people with disabilities in their chapter, "Chemical Dependency: The Avoided Issue for Persons with Physical Disabilities." They discuss issues which may perpetuate chemical dependency in people with disabilities, myths about substance abuse and disabilities, responses by family and friends which may enable substance use, and describe how professionals can assist in clients' pursuit of substance abuse services. They describe their model chemical dependence program at Abbott Northwestern Hospital and the Sister Kinney Institute for persons with physical disabilities, the philosophy which guides treatment, the way in which the program is staffed, and the outcomes achieved by the program.

Linda Cherry describes how a grassroots effort led to the building of a coalition between professionals and consumers who were concerned about substance abuse by persons with physical disabilities. Her chapter, "Institute on Alcohol, Drugs, and Disability: From Grassroots Activity to Systems Changes," describes the steps taken by a voluntary group of providers and consumers to survey needs and services in their region, and the results of two surveys. For the first time, they compiled service statistics from chemical dependence treatment programs describing the extent to which disability concerns were addressed and clients with disabilities were served. The results of a second survey in which disability service agencies were questioned about the ways in which they deal with alcohol and other drug issues are also reported. Training issues and recommendations are proposed to better serve the chemical dependence treatment needs of persons with disabilities.

The next chapter in this section, "Comprehensive Treatment of Addictive Families" by Stephen Schlesinger and Lawrence Horberg, summarizes a developmental model of family recovery from addiction. The authors describe system-specific features of the model and then consider application of the model to persons with disabilities. The model describes treatment as a journey from chaos to family health and attempts to engage all interested members. Stages of exasperation, effort, and empowerment are described, and specific ways in which therapists can assist families on this journey are detailed.

The concluding chapter in this section, "Evaluating Treatment Services" by Thomas Budziack, highlights ways in which rehabilitation professionals can deal effectively with a variety of barriers to help clients with disabilities receive appropriate treatment for substance abuse. He describes how to request a thorough and complete assessment, evaluate substance abuse treatment providers and their services, and refer clients to treatment that is well matched to their needs. He reviews various types of treatment sources and providers, lists questions to ask of assessors and service providers, describes strategies to determine the appropriate treatment intensity, and how to develop substance abuse services for clients with disabilities when none are available.

The summary section, comprised of a single chapter, "Issues and Controversies in Chemical Dependence Services for Persons with

Physical Disabilities" by Deborah Kiley and Michael Brandt, highlights issues that emerge from earlier discussions of chemical dependence and disability topics. They discuss chemical dependence issues which directly impact persons with disabilities in terms of prevention, assessment, and treatment. Client issues, such as inaccessible treatment service and legitimate access to abusable prescription medications, system issues, such as the paucity of treatment services which are sensitive to disability issues, and research issues, such as the dearth of outcome studies, are also reviewed.

Rehabilitation and chemical dependence professionals can be effective partners in serving the needs of clients with disabilities and substance abuse problems. Enhancing prevention and treatment services will require engaging independent living centers, consumer advocacy groups such as the National Head Injury Foundation, the National Spinal Cord Injury Association and their state affiliates, and state vocational and substance abuse agencies, as well as professionals in a variety of disciplines. This text is intended to address important and timely issues, such as mainstreaming disability issues within the chemical dependence field, and including substance abuse services as a legitimate issue within rehabilitation settings. The obvious next steps are to incorporate alcohol and other drug abuse education within rehabilitation professionals' training, and disability topics within chemical dependence professionals' curricula. Clearly these two groups have a common agenda: enhancing the independence of all individuals and promoting the development of lifestyles which demonstrate a positive regard for one's health and well-being. The development of more integrated and responsive service systems will entail a shared perspective by rehabilitation and chemical dependence professionals which is holistic in structure and requires unique expertise.

Chapter 2

Addicted and Disabled:
One Man's Journey
from Helplessness to Hope

Kenneth K. Gorman, CAC-1

It wasn't until a year ago that I remembered what happened in my accident. I knew I was drinking, but over the years I had invented a story about hitting a patch of ice and sliding off the highway. The truth is, I was drunk. It was about 3:00 a.m. and I had been drinking nearly all day. I was supposed to report for work at 7:00 a.m. in a small town in Colorado. I was pouring a drink and I lost the cap to the bottle somewhere in the car. I took my eyes off the road to look for the cap. It seemed that I looked away only a moment, but when you're drunk a moment can be three minutes. My Volkswagen jerked and rolled and I thought, "Oh God, I've done it. I pushed it to the limit this time." I remember a gnawing in my gut and wondering, "Will I survive this one?" The feeling was familiar, that "living on the edge" feeling, I had felt so many times in the past. I was raised in a dysfunctional family where there were no boundaries. One day I could do something and it was all right and the next day I could do the same exact thing and I was punished for it. Over the years it created a lot of confusion and a feeling of walking on eggshells with others in my family; that is where a lot of my thrill seeking-personality comes from. Basically I became very addicted to that feeling; although I didn't like it much, I had to have it. When I took my first drink at eight years of age I found the alcohol made the "on edge" feeling comfortable and manageable. The alcohol made me feel like I fit in a world where I felt I hadn't fit before. It was like magic; when I took a drink I felt calmness and serenity within. My point of view, and the point of view of many other recovering alcoholics, is that drugs and alcohol are a symptom of my inability to manage my own life. Alcohol did this for me–it gave me control over my emotions; it eliminated the fear so that I had the courage to be myself.

The Volkswagen came to a stop. I realized I had just driven off a cliff. I remember being upside down and feeling my back hurt a little. I pulled my body free from the car, paralyzing myself. I was a long way from the highway, and it was dark and cold, but I felt a sense of relief. I was out of the competition, it was over, the hell I was living in was over. I knew either I would die or be taken care of, and I fell asleep not caring whether I lived or died.

A noise woke me up. It was somebody moving a rock. The sun was shining but I was shivering. I looked at the sun: "About 8:00," I thought. A woman walked up to me and covered me with her coat. She said, "Don't move, the helicopter is on its way." I remember a lot of confusion and a lot of people were standing over me. It kind of reminded me of the movies when somebody passes out and they wake up and all they see are faces bending over. The helicopter came, they put me on it, and the first thing I asked for was something for the pain. Because I was quite hung over I didn't have much pain but there was something haunting me and that was what I had just done to myself. I knew what would fix that haunting feeling–more dope. I knew doctors had good dope; all addicts know that. It is all spiked up and ready to go. I didn't have to go through the hassle of cooking it up. It was March 21, 1981, a date I will never forget.

One day my father walked into my hospital room and asked, "Are you finally going to do something?" He was referring to my alcoholism and drug addiction. I told him I didn't want to hear it. I was on a path to self-destruction; I didn't want help. The loss of both my legs was not even enough to make me give up my drugs and alcohol. My friends smuggled booze to me in the intensive care unit at the hospital. I watched the clock waiting for my morphine shot every three hours. I didn't have much pain, but I liked the morphine high. Pain was an excuse to get high and I used it. A doctor at the rehabilitation hospital asked if I liked beer. I told him, "No, but I like hard liquor every once in a while." So he wrote in my chart that I could drink while in rehabilitation. (I remember how he wrote it . . . "Let Ken have his spirits.")

I told people I didn't want cards or flowers, so they sent bottles of liquor. Mixing the liquor with the pain medication was wonderful. I didn't have to deal with my grief over the loss of my legs. They could have cut off my arms and I wouldn't have cared. It was interesting that no one ever confronted me on my alcoholism when in rehabilitation; I remember not only was I justifying my alcoholism by getting off the pain medication but it seemed the doctors were also. I can remember them telling me how well I was doing in weaning myself off the pain medication. Actually it was quite easy because I was just replacing it with alcohol. I very much got the impression that it was not only I who didn't want to admit that I had a problem, neither did the doctors. After all if the doctors admitted that I had a problem, it would have been their obligation to do something about it and at that time there were no resources for dealing with disability and substance abuse. Something else I believe played into it was the fact that my doctor was an alcoholic himself.

I got out of rehabilitation six weeks later. I didn't have a high school education. I couldn't go back to my job with the railroad and the only other work I had done was tending bar and knocking heads. I wasn't interested in going back to school, so I turned to what I knew best–the street–conning and manipulating people for drugs and money. I fell into what I call wheelchair games and I'm not talking the Wheelchair Olympics; I found that the wheelchair gave me powerful access to others' sympathy and I played on that sympathy enough to support a $300.00 a day drug habit.

It was three years later that I was sitting in a vacant warehouse. I had been there for nine months. I had a .38 caliber pistol in my mouth and was ready to blow my brains all over the ceiling. At that time my total assets were an old, stainless wheelchair that was falling apart, a pair of 501s, a pair of Converse All-Star tennis shoes, and a .38 which was in my mouth. I had no place to live, no food, no money, no friends. I had been stabbed and shot in numerous drug wars. I had stolen and conned money from my friends by playing on their pity and guilt. I was kicked out of most of the bars in town for hustling pool, gambling, or just being obnoxious. It got to the point where the dealers wouldn't even sell to me anymore. One dealer told me, "You are killing yourself, man. I ain't selling you no more drugs." So there I was with numerous skin sores, a bladder infection, a 12" by 3" burn on my leg from shooting hot dope–ready to blow my brains out. I was beat; it had won. I remember thinking, "Is this it? Is this the only reason I've been put on earth? To die like this?" And then I prayed to God, "Please, help me. Whether I pull the trigger or not, please, help me." I heard a radio in the distance. A song was playing that I had heard before, but this time I listened and the answer came. I couldn't give up yet. I knew of a drug and alcohol treatment center. They had refused me before but I decided to try one more time. I called the treatment center and talked with them for awhile, telling them where I was and what I was about to do. They said they would have somebody call me back. I thought, "Sure, you will," and hung up. The phone rang; it was the treatment center. They were sending a cab for me. That was October 30, 1984. I have been clean ever since.

I was angry when I decided to quit drugs and alcohol. I was angry at reality. But most of all I was angry at myself. I was angry for drugging. It was my responsibility; no one else was to blame, not even God. It was the most difficult thing I had to own. If I had admitted that I was responsible for the things that had happened, I would have been admitting a problem with alcohol and drugs, and that was the last thing I wanted to do. I was also very self-centered. I didn't do anything unless there was something in it for me. My whole life was centered around drugs and alcohol. Either I was doing drugs and alcohol, or getting ready to do drugs and alcohol, or thinking of ways to get money to do drugs and alcohol and in the process I hurt a lot of people. After all, it's very difficult to watch somebody destroy his life the way I did.

I was in complete denial about my feelings and emotions. Feeling like a child, everyone was an authority figure to me. I had no views or values. I felt as though in my 25 years nothing had been accomplished but self-destruction. I was beat. I had had it! Drugs and alcohol had won again, just as they had won many times in the past.

The bottom line was fear. I was scared of failure. I was afraid of success. I was afraid of living and I was afraid of death. Although suicidal thoughts stayed with me once I had become sober, I even used that as a tool to stay sober. I was through with drugs and alcohol and I figured "if it gets much worse, I will just kill myself." But the funny thing was that as long as I didn't take a drink or drugs, it never got any worse; it slowly got better and better. The logic being I was not willing to go through the slow suicide of alcoholism and drug addiction.

I awoke to the fact that substance abuse is a symptom, that all of the reasons above were the main reasons I used. It wasn't so much that I had a problem with drugs and alcohol, I had a problem with life and accepting life on life's terms. I would go to any lengths to escape reality; I was addicted to escaping reality–as many people are. People are addicted to television, to eating, to sex, drugs, and rock and roll. I was, and am, one of those people. After seven years of being clean and sober, I am still just one drink away from losing everything. There's a saying that when you get hit by a train, it's not the caboose that kills you. So, I do not take the first drink. I had a thousand excuses to continue using, but not one to sober up. I used to love drizzly days, because it instantly gave me an excuse to get drunk or high. Sunny days were great too, because it was such a gorgeous day to enjoy a drink in the sun.

I surrendered and was ready to quit. The bottom line is, I wanted to help myself. I was willing to go to any lengths to stay free of drugs and alcohol, just as I had been willing to go to any lengths to get high. I figured that I could put at least the same amount of energy into staying sober as I did into getting high. I recognized that I had a disease, that it wasn't my fault, but that it was my responsibility to do something about it. I believe in the disease concept of alcoholism and drug addiction; in psychological and physical addiction to drugs–the self-centered, sick behavior, when drugs and alcohol become the most important thing in life, before family, friends, and taking care of ourselves and life's responsibilities. My disability became an excuse for my alcoholism and drug addiction. Not only did it become an excuse for me, but also for my peers. I remember many times going to the bar and getting pats on the back, and people saying, " It's good to see people like you out having a good time." I viewed the bar as a way of working myself back into society. The belief that I drank because of my disability was ludicrous; I was a full-fledged drunk before I became disabled. My alcoholism and drug addiction did not emerge from my disability, my disability emerged from my alcoholism and drug addiction.

I now belong to a twelve-step fellowship program that has helped a great deal in my recovery from alcoholism and drug addiction. For a long time I wondered why I was the way I was; now I know. The only way I got the answers I needed was through complete abstinence and self-honesty. It wasn't easy at first, but it gets easier all the time. The chatter that was in my head went away after awhile, and the peacefulness I feel now is wonderful. On the street I was always running from myself. I don't have to do that anymore. When I was running, I didn't like me much. Today, I love myself a lot. Today, I have friends, real friends who love me and I love them.

My reality today is I can't take drugs. Not even medicine prescribed by a doctor. I remember having a network of doctors who were all very quick to medicate; it seemed that all I had to do was mention pain or spasms and they wrote me a prescription. I sold most of my prescription drugs or traded them for street drugs or alcohol. I finally realized that I couldn't fix things with a pill anymore. I had to find ways of dealing with phantom pain, so I learned self-hypnosis. A lot of medical complications went away when I stopped drinking (spasms, bladder infections, skin sores, stab and gunshot wounds, etc.). At about six months the leg spasms went away. I learned that the alcohol I had been drinking stimulated the nerves and caused the spasms. I haven't had a skin sore since going clean. When I got drunk or high I wouldn't move, so I got sores.

Today I am free, free from the addiction, and in being free I have opportunities. The only opportunity I had before was to stick a needle in my arm every day and be a slave to a drug or die. Those were my options, I thought. Today I am in college and make a nice living as an addictions therapist.

I feel I need to mention the importance of relationships—friendships as well as intimate relationships. As I began my recovery, for a long time I couldn't allow someone to love me. If somebody wanted to do something for me, I would instantly ask myself, "What do they want?" It felt like a set-up. You see, the street is a place where everybody takes advantage of everybody else. If I help you on the street and you accept that help, you instantly owe me. And every time we look at each other we both know it. I had to come to terms with the fact that everyone needs help, not just the handicapped. It wasn't easy letting somebody help me, but I did it. Today I can give love and receive love without any expectations. I am totally grateful for who I am and what I am. I thank God for giving me the opportunity to reach out and help another human being, no matter who or what they are. Today I am in a relationship with a wonderful woman whom I love very much. I want to live and continue living. It is not easy sometimes, but we need to hold our heads up and endure. We need to move forward instead of hiding out from life. We need to start looking at what we have instead of what we don't have.

Each year, 10,000 to 15,000 people in the United States become spinal cord injured. Fifty thousand people a year survive disabling head injuries. A spinal cord injury or the loss of cognitive functioning is difficult to cope with. Such an injury can shatter every aspect of one's life, and the feelings of loss and anger can be all-consuming. The person with a disability may feel that life as a whole human being is over. Subsequently, feelings of inadequacy, low self-esteem, and lack of confidence surface with full force. This is further complicated by feelings of desperation and loneliness; the individual with a disability will often become isolated and drink or use other drugs. He or she is unable to accept disability and will avoid reality at all costs. The person is also unable to accept the consequences of his or her disability. For example, a number of individuals, after acquiring a disability, experience sexual dysfunction. This situation creates feelings of sexual inadequacy and fear of the opposite sex. As the individual with a disability quietly suffers he or she turns to alcohol and drugs to mask the intensity of feelings.

Another consequence of disability may be the inability to return to work. A large number of individuals with disabilities lack a college education and in many cases lack a high school education. Thus, many were previously employed in blue collar positions. Once injured, the individual is unable to return to his or her prior employment and is now faced with a questionable future, limited career options, and no vocational direction. The task of vocational rehabilitation is overwhelming and the person turns to alcohol and other drugs.

Not only does substance abuse show up as a coping mechanism

after an injury, but oftentimes there is a pre-existing substance problem prior to an injury. An alarming number of these injuries, 62%, can be attributed to taking unnecessary risks while under the influence of alcohol and drugs. This self-destructive behavior continues to be manifested after an individual acquires a disability and his tendency to use is impacted further. It is also important to note that oftentimes the medical profession is too quick to medicate acute and chronic pain. In many cases, professionals support addictions by supplying drugs without investigating pre-existing substance problems.

In my experience, I have noted three major difficulties in addressing substance abuse among persons with spinal cord and head injuries. First, a number of these individuals are recipients of Social Security benefits and are covered by Medicaid or Medicare. Unfortunately, if an individual with a disability is chemically dependent, treatment options are limited. Medicare will pay for 21 days of in-hospital treatment and will not cover outpatient counseling. Medicaid will not pay for either and makes little attempt to address a substance problem. The second difficulty is that a number of alcohol and drug treatment centers are not adequately equipped to deal with individuals who have disabilities. There are too many physical barriers and treatment personnel generally are not educated and experienced in disability issues. Often an inability exists to break through the emotional barrier the disabled individual has built to protect himself or herself. Further, most rehabilitation workers have not addressed their own understanding and values regarding disability issues. Often the disabled individual himself or herself is unable to break through the emotional barrier that has been built for protection.

Third, even if an individual with a disability gets into treatment he or she often fails within one to two months of treatment. The reasons for this are many:

1. If the disability was not addressed in treatment, the obstacles to be faced in aftercare will not be addressed. These obstacles include transportation to Alcoholics Anonymous and Narcotics Anonymous meetings, accessibility, and appropriate outpa-

tient counseling to deal with substance abuse and disability issues.

2. Frequently, insurance money runs out or Medicare monies are no longer available.
3. Many return to unhealthy living environments which threaten their sobriety.
4. A number of individuals are unaware of the resources available to them, including state's divisions of rehabilitation.
5. Because a number of persons with disabilities are unemployed, there is a significant amount of time on their hands once discharged, and an inability to fulfill leisure time needs.
6. Institutionalization provides a number of disabled individuals who have substance abuse problems with a comfortable environment which allows them to relive dysfunctional family issues from their past.
7. The rehabilitation environment itself can be dysfunctional. A number of individuals from dysfunctional families go into the caretaking professions such as nursing, counseling, and psychology. This creates dysfunctional roles for the patient and professional.

Three years ago I started an outpatient program called Helping Handicapped Addictions With Knowledge (H.H.A.W.K.) which is designed to address these issues in multidisabled, substance abusers. H.H.A.W.K., Inc. is a private, nonprofit organization which consists of a Board of Directors, a volunteer counselor, and a bookkeeper/secretary. I serve as the Executive Director and have been substance-free for five years. I am an alcohol and drug counselor certified by the state of Colorado. Our volunteer, Stephen Hahn, in his second year of freedom from chemical dependency, has a developmental disability and is working on certification through the state of Colorado. Stephen is also a graduate of H.H.A.W.K., Inc. The program provides a number of services. We counsel in all areas of addiction. In addition, we provide Adult Children of Alcoholics (A.C.O.A.), with sexuality, peer and dysfunctional family counseling, and education. Our organization consults and designs programs for rehabilitation facilities. We also work with a number of hospitals and other institutions in addressing substance abuse in the rehabilitation environment.

Recently we have begun to plan adding a speaker's program to our services. We were contacted by the Colorado Governor's Office and Communities for a Drug Free Colorado to help prevent substance abuse and driving. A number of individuals who have successfully maintained their lives without the use of drugs or alcohol, all of whom were involved in serious accidents, have rehearsed their presentations. The experience has allowed them to grow considerably in their recovery. We plan to make this program part of therapy. Not only do the speakers grow, but we are giving back to the community in several ways: (1) prevention of spinal cord and head injuries that result from drinking or drugging and driving, (2) education on disability awareness, (3) education on wearing seat belts, and (4) education on responsible drinking or drug use, if individuals choose to use them. We will speak to businesses, churches, schools, rehabilitation institutions, and addiction treatment centers.

As I continue to work with addicts with disabilities I find that my story is not unique. My pain and frustration was as an individual who could not accept his alcoholism and drug addiction. What I needed to do first was accept my addiction over the years. All the rehabilitation in the world would be unsuccessful until I addressed the issue of substance abuse in my life. As professionals in rehabilitation it is our responsibility to address issues concerning our own lives before we can begin to address others' issues. It is also our responsibility to understand that we cannot ignore the problem of substance abuse among persons with disabilities any longer.

Chapter 3

A Personological Integration of Chemical Dependence and Physical Disability

Franklin C. Shontz, PhD

This chapter is about rehabilitation, but not about the kind of rehabilitation that most people are likely to think of immediately. It is not about the rehabilitation of decrepit houses or of decaying neighborhoods in large cities. Nor is it about head injuries, cardiac conditions or any particular forms of disability, physical or otherwise. Nevertheless, the subject matter of this chapter should arouse considerable interest among professionals who are involved in helping people who suffer misfortune of any kind.

Although this chapter is surely concerned with the rehabilitation of human beings, it is more directly concerned with the rehabilitation of a too-long neglected scientific method, the case study. The chapter attempts to demonstrate how the rehabilitation of that method can eventually lead to considerable improvement in the concepts and practices that guide service provision to persons in many kinds of settings.

HOLISM

This chapter is not about holism as such, but a brief discussion of that concept may serve a useful introductory purpose. For several years the word holism has enjoyed considerable popularity and has influenced theory and practice in several helping professions, including rehabilitation. The term was coined in 1926 by Jan Smuts, a famous South African statesman and soldier, in a book titled *Holism and Evolution*. The word holism is derived from the Greek root *holos*, meaning complete, whole, entire.

The holistic point of view was most thoroughly espoused by Kurt Goldstein, who used it in 1939 in the title of his book, *The Organism: A Holistic Approach to Biology Derived from Pathological Data in Men*. Goldstein was concerned with proposing a solution to the mind body problem based on his observations of persons who had suffered brain injuries in war (Goldstein, 1942). He also studied psychopathology, especially schizophrenia. In 1940 he published a comprehensive treatise, *Human Nature in the Light of Psychopathology* (Goldstein, 1940) in which he applied his holistic, or organismic, viewpoint to understand individual development and to underscore the responsibilities of society to promote the self-actualization (Goldstein's word) of its members. Holistic ideas and the concept of self-actualization have also become familiar through the personality theories of Carl Rogers and Abraham Maslow.

HOLISM AND REHABILITATION

In the context of a consideration of the principles of rehabilitation, two features of the holistic/organismic approach require special emphasis. The first is its implication that the primary concern in developing a plan for patient care is not the person's physical condition as such. Rather, the primary task is to determine the part that the physical state of the person plays in his or her life as a whole. The second is that, although apparent disturbances or deficits in a person's behavior are usually thought of as being symptomatic of specific physical pathologies, they are not what they seem to be. They are not disturbances of behavior but reasonable strategies that the person adopts in order to cope as effectively as possible with the person's life situation, as that person understands it. A possible exception occurs in a state called the catastrophic reaction. This is a condition of complete disorganization that takes over when the total personal structure of the individual collapses and becomes chaotic.

According to the organismic point of view, jargon aphasia, for example, is not to be viewed as a symptom of disorders in the fibers that connect specific areas of the brain. Rather, it is the best possible effort on the part of the person to communicate, given the conditions under which that person must function. In rehabilitation, the holistic/organismic position shifts the conceptual emphasis from trying to figure out what is wrong with the person so that the defect can be corrected, to considering what the organism as a whole is trying to accomplish and how the organism can be helped to do it better. The holistic/organismic view does not see the task of professional care to be diagnosing and curing pathologies or correcting physical defects. Instead, it proposes a truly rehabilitative philosophy. It calls for maximizing individual potential by enhancing adaptive possibilities and discovering new capabilities, within the limits imposed by a given set of organismic states or processes.

One consequence of the holistic/organismic way of thinking is that it necessitates becoming increasingly concerned about promoting the welfare of all aspects of individual client's lives. It is not enough to regard someone's rehabilitation as being complete merely because the person has learned how to avoid skin breakdowns and function in a wheelchair. To the extent that modern rehabilitation is holistic, it concerns itself as well with what effect living in a wheelchair will have on that person's vocational adjustment, social life, self-esteem, and emotional state. The modern rehabilitation worker should not only know a great deal about specific physical or psychiatric conditions but should also be prepared to apply that knowledge in the context of an understanding of the life situation of each client who is treated.

The well-known team approach evolved primarily in response to recognition of the fact that every client brings to rehabilitation a unique combination of physical, mental, interpersonal, and social conditions, all of which must be taken into account in the development of treatment plans and in the performance of outcome evaluations. That is to say that the philosophy of modern rehabilitation, if not always its actual practice, has not only implicitly accepted the basic principle of holism, but it has also, of necessity, become increasingly individualized and, as some would say it, personological.

Kenneth Gorman's story, in the preceding chapter, shows how

revealing and how moving a penetrating look into the life of an individual human being can be. His story is revealing because it describes as no other type of exposition can how a disability fits into a whole life situation; how intricately interwoven drug use, life style, self-concept and physical disability are; some of the psychological conditions that must be met if rehabilitation is to be lastingly effective; and how the process of adapting to disability can be a transformative personal experience. His story is moving because it exposes how powerfully the entire process of adaptation is driven by emotion from start to finish. That is especially important because workers in rehabilitation often shy away from or try not to be affected by the intense emotional reactions of many of their clients.

Mr. Gorman says that his story is not unique, and the reader intuitively recognizes that he is correct. But of course his story is not generalizable to every single drug user or to every single person with a physical disability either. What the serious scientist or practitioner wants to know is which aspects of Mr. Gorman's experience belong to him alone, which are true of drug and alcohol users in general (whether they have disabilities or not), which apply to all persons with disabilities (whether they are or are not drug and alcohol users), and which are universal in the sense that they apply to everyone, because all human beings must sooner or later face defeat, pain, suffering and the prospect of death. To gain such knowledge requires adopting a systematic approach, not only to narratives that are produced spontaneously by persons like Kenneth Gorman, but to the entire process of research design, data collection, and interpretation and analysis of results. This is the mission of scientific method, and more particularly it is the task that must be completed if the case study method is to achieve the rehabilitation it so rightly deserves.

THE PERSONOLOGIC PERSPECTIVE

Personology may be thought of as an attempt to apply the principles of holism to the systematic study and treatment of human beings, considered one at a time. It examines individual people in all their complexity, rather than as representatives of diagnostic categories or as deviants from norms on measures of specific factors or characteristics. Personology does not require adopting any particular theory. It is a method, a way of gaining scientifically useful information from individual persons without minimizing their complexity or denying their distinctively human characteristics. With regard to substance abuse, for example, a conventional research project might compare the means of large samples of drug users and nonusers on a psychological test of depression to determine whether the groups as wholes differ significantly. A personological study would examine several individual drug users intensively and extensively to learn how and why each became involved in drug use and what part drug use plays in the lives of each one of them. Similarly, with regard to the effects of a condition such as spinal cord injury, personological research would examine closely, both in breadth and in depth, as many aspects as possible of the lives and experiences of particular individuals who have spinal cord injuries, in order to learn how their conditions affect each one of them.

The personological approach need not be limited to carrying out naturalistic and nonintervening descriptions of situations or individuals. It has considerable potential in both treatment and evaluation programs (Shontz, 1988). For example, instead of using a single, uniform standard that is applied uniformly to clients indiscriminately at the end-point of therapy, assessment of treatment effectiveness can be carried out longitudinally, in terms of the success of achievement of goals that are personalized along dimensions relevant to each individual (see, for example, Korchin & Schuldberg, 1981).

In 1938, H.A. Murray proposed that the term *personology* be used to refer to "the branch of psychology which principally concerns the study of human lives and the factors that influence their course . . ." (Murray, 1938, p. 4). Murray did not work in the field of rehabilitation of persons with physical disabilities, so his theory does not stress the functional significance of most forms of physical handicap. Rather, it emphasizes motivational forces or drives which are called needs, social and environmental forces which are called presses, and cognitive or ideational processes, which are called themes. Personology need not be identified specifically with psychology, as Murray proposed. It is available for use by people in any discipline that deals with human functioning.

The word personology is easily misused. For example, a recent review of the literature on the relationship between personality and addiction (Sutker & Allain, 1988) concludes that the postulation of such a relationship is, in essence, simplistic. In that review the authors appear to equate personology with psychoanalytic theory, and that is an unwarranted oversimplification. The authors adopted a stance toward research on alcohol and drug use that they described as "a conceptual schemata (sic) that encompasses multifactorial, reciprocal and integrative explanations of the etiology, natural history, and progression of addictive disorders and their comorbidities" (p. 172). Yet, the review neglects to suggest that the best way to study drug use within such schemata is obviously through the intensive examination of individuals, studied one at time.

The goal of personological study is not to understand every conceivable aspect of any individual human being. The purpose of personological study is to understand the relevant aspects of each individual, where relevance is determined, as it is in all scientific research, by the question that is asked of the data that are eventually collected. For example, if an investigator were to study how one person manages the anticipation, experience of and recovery from surgery to examine and remove malignant tissue in the kidneys, detailed medical data would be as important as information about the person's feelings or vocational and family situation and life plans. Hesitation about regarding such a study as belonging strictly to a branch of psychology would certainly be justified. Putting questions of professional identity and semantics aside, however, this hypothetical example makes one point clear. It is that the stock in trade of the personological approach is the case study, and not the usual forms of large scale sociological epidemiological surveys or statistical comparisons of selected groups. These more conventional methods serve important purposes in rehabilitation-relevant research, and they will continue to do so. But they usually do not tell rehabilitation professionals who work in service settings what they usually want to know in practice. That is: Why does this particular client act in this particular way, and what can I do to help?

Most rehabilitation professionals who work with clients one at a time do not learn how to answer questions like these by reading textbooks or by examining reports of research that has been carried out in laboratories or on large groups of subjects. They may, of course, recall having read about a similar case, but by and large they answer such questions by referring to acquired experiences with similar clients in the past. These experiences may be their own, as when a therapist says, "The last time I had a client like this . . . ," or they may be someone else's, as when a supervisor says, "In cases like this, we usually find that . . ." Only when such referral to experience fails is the therapist likely to call upon another professional, a clinical psychologist, for example, for additional specialized help. The trouble with this way of answering important questions in the treatment setting is that it is unsystematic. It fails to meet the standards of science in three ways. First, it is not objective, because it does not carefully document observations or measure phenomena in reliable ways.

Second, it does not produce cumulative public knowledge. The knowledge it produces is cumulative only in the limited sense that each individual therapist gains personal knowledge with each case. It is not public, however, because so little of the therapist's knowledge is made available to others, either in complete form as an archive or in condensed form as a set of summarized recommendations that others can test for themselves.

Lack of accessibility of knowledge to others leads to the third failure, which is that the knowledge is not open to criticism. It is therefore not amenable to correction through the enhancement process that takes place when attempts are made to reply to logical objections or to answer empirical questions by collecting more data in new or improved ways. The point is that, if these limitations are overcome, properly conducted case studies can be a valuable source of information and knowledge. They can contribute a great deal not only to increasing the scientific understanding of persons but to the improvement of treatment strategies and evaluation techniques.

REPRESENTATIVE CASE RESEARCH

The results of a study using a specific approach to personological research, called the Representative Case Method, are described below. In Representative Case Research a particular individual is selected or recruited for examination because he or she has special knowledge that qualifies him or her to act as an expert consultant on a topic that is of particular interest to the investigator. Unlike many case studies, Representative Case Research is carefully planned in advance and designed to answer specific questions in systematic ways. Some examples of Representative Case Research are a series of nine case studies of individual chronic, heavy users of cocaine, published by James Spotts and Franklin Shontz (1980). A more recent example is a case study by Jennifer Gordon and Franklin Shontz of a young man who tested positive for the AIDS virus but was asymptomatic (1990a). Specifics about how such research may be carried out are described in another article by Gordon and Shontz (1990b) in a subsequent issue of the same journal (*Journal of Counseling and Development*).

Representative case studies, which concern persons with spinal cord injuries, are the studies of two persons that were conducted by Heinemann and Shontz on the topic of adjustment following physical disability (Heinemann & Shontz, 1984). In this research, the investigators examined in systematic fashion the roles that two individuals with very different rehabilitation outcomes felt disability played in their lives. In order to obtain normative data about the characteristics of these people, both were first given standard tests of intelligence and personality. They were then asked to examine their life histories and to choose several critical episodes, which served as reference points for further study. Spontaneous and guided imagery were used to induce reexperiencing of these episodes, and several specially developed psychological measuring techniques were administered after every reexperiencing to assess each person's reactions to the episodes.

The results of these studies highlighted the importance of previously established coping styles as well as of the environment in shaping adjustment to disability. One person (Deirdre), whose life had always been inner-directed, showed the theoretically expected psychological stages of emotional adjustment to her condition, but the stages did not occur in the predicted order. Furthermore, they did not appear spontaneously, as theory might suggest, but were usually triggered by external events. The other person (Craig) was not at all introspective and denied having experienced depression or having undergone any noticeable changes in his emotional state as a result of his disability.

Both of these persons were making satisfactory behavioral adjustments at the time of the studies, although Craig had previously attempted suicide. That attempt, he said, was not a response to depression but an attempt to regain control over his existence. Craig's data seemed to show that adequate behavioral adaptation to life crisis may sometimes occur even in the absence of an awareness that one is working through intense personal reactions. However, the data also seemed to show that some rather extreme form of felt or behaviorally expressed response, whether or not it is accompanied by the conscious experience of depression, may be necessary if personal growth is to take place following the occurrence of profound life crisis.

The data on the individual who is to be discussed in more detail here come from another series of Representative Case Studies of chronic, heavy drug users. These were carried out by James Spotts and myself and were studies of amphetamine users. This report is presented in narrative form, but the report is derived from the close examination of extensive and intensive data derived from structured and unstructured interviews, normed tests of cognitive functioning and personality, Q-sorts, Rep-Test grids and special techniques devised specifically for the research program.

THE CASE OF DON J.

The person of interest is a man who will be called Don J. At the time he was examined, Don was 44 years old. He was mobile in a wheelchair, having been paralyzed about 20 years previously by a spinal cord injury that was sustained as a result of an automobile accident. Though not a large man, Don was muscular and lean, with the sort of physique that might be described as wiry. He spoke willingly on all topics but was always acutely conscious of the impression he was making. Don was not genuinely insightful, but he felt confident about his self-knowledge and he was adept at convincing any listener of his sincerity.

As part of his participation in this research, Don was examined with a battery of standardized, normed psychological tests, as well as with objective measures that were individually tailored to assess important features of his life. He was exhaustively interviewed about his personal past, especially his history of drug use. He was asked to name every substance he could remember having used and to respond to check lists to describe the physiological and psychological reactions he experienced when taking each. Similar procedures were employed for each of the other eight persons in the series of amphetamines users and for nine matched persons in each of five other groups, four of which contained users of cocaine, opiates, barbiturates and sedative-hypnotics, and PCP, and one of which contained a group of comparable persons who had been exposed to drugs but had determined not to use them. The data on which this description of Don J. is based were obtained in 1977. They were collected at the Greater Kansas City Mental Health Foundation in Kansas City, Missouri, and my colleague, James V. Spotts, who was the Assistant Director of that organization, deserves the credit for undertaking the task of collecting most of them.

While reading this description of Don J., bear in mind that our reason for studying this man was not to check the validity of his statements or to question the accuracy of his reports. Nor were we concerned with his medical condition or his rehabilitation as such. The goal of the study was to gain insight into Don's experiences, particularly those that are drug related, not to criticize him. The study could be called phenomenological, at least in part, because among other things its purpose was to enable the investigators to see the world and Don's life as much as possible as he saw it. For example, Don admitted that he used drugs, particularly amphetamines for most of his life. In describing his reasons for doing so, he said in effect that he once took amphetamines for pleasure and to support his defiant life style. Now (that is, at the time of the research), he says his primary reason for using amphetamines is that they reduce the muscle spasms and pain associated with his physical disability, and they give him the energy he needs to keep going in the face of recurrent depression. He is convinced that amphetamines are more efficacious and less dangerous than opiates or barbiturates, to which he says he has been addicted in the past. He believes that many other paraplegics and quadriplegics could be helped if physicians would only give amphetamines a fair test. As researchers studying persons we did not see it as our task to question the genuineness of Don's beliefs, opinions or experiences, nor is this material presented to make his argument for him. No doubt Don would be overjoyed if he knew that he was the subject of this chapter, but I am not at all certain that he would feel his case for the use of amphetamines as medication is being adequately advanced.

Formal Testing

On the Wechsler Adult Intelligence Scale, Don evidenced a high level of verbal intelligence and a comparatively low level of ability on performance tests. He was especially bothered by the tests that placed heavy demands upon speed of performance, and the effects of his disability clearly interfered with some of his movements on these tests. Although his overall IQ was about average for the normative population of his age, Don was found to possess a very good vocabulary, a high level of capacity for abstraction and good comprehension of social norms and expectations.

His MMPI record showed him to be a person who uses rather sophisticated personal defenses, who is sensitive to others but who is at the same time extremely rebellious, even antisocial, and who is prone to display his own feelings in dramatic ways. Also apparent on the MMPI was considerable anxiety and concern over somatic symptoms. There was evidence in the test profile that he typically operates at a high energy level, but the record gave no reason to suspect the presence of serious schizophrenic or other psychotic mental processes.

On the Sixteen Personality Factors Questionnaire, which is a test designed to measure normal traits of personality, Don J. described himself as being imaginative and venturesome, forthright, unpretentious and practical. He acknowledged a tendency to ignore social conventions and also said that he is emotionally unstable, changeable, and easily upset.

On other tests of personality factors, he described himself as being a person who loves to take risks and be in dangerous situations. He seeks out novelty, dislikes routines and is intolerant of monotony. On Q-sort measures of self concept, his data were inconsistent from one occasion to the next. He typically denied having negative personality traits, and he constantly tried to present a positive image of himself. He revealed a preference for acting decisively, but he also admitted a somewhat contrary tendency to act impulsively. One might suppose that Don J. is a good representative of the group of high risk taking individuals who are rather prominently represented in the population of persons with spinal cord injuries. On the Role Repertory Test, he showed a strong desire to be at peace with himself, but this wish was coupled with a basic distrust of others. Don seemed to be trying to convince himself that he is self sufficient, independent and not tied down to anyone. Yet, he seemed also to be wishing to be able to find the peace he desires by relating to someone who will play the role of the strong, dependable loving father for him. The wish has turned out to be self-defeating, because Don has spent a lifetime convincing himself that no one, especially anyone with authority over him, is to be trusted.

Life History

Don's childhood was spent in a large midwestern city. His father was an alcoholic, and although he held jobs from time to time, he squandered most of his money on drink and gambling. When Don was a child he would accompany his father to the taverns and listen to the people talk. That is when he felt closest to his father. He describes his mother as being loving and affectionate, but easy to con, and Don remembers that he conned her all the time. The first time that Don was picked up by the police she "raised hell" with Don's father, because in her opinion he should have been watching out for the boy and never should have let it happen. Don has a younger brother and an older sister but is not close to either of them and apparently never has been.

Don began working during the Second World War. He was about twelve years old at the time, and there were not many men around to do the work. He washed dishes in a restaurant, set pins in a bowling alley, and picked up golf balls at a driving range; he also learned to gamble. He claims that he was basically self-sufficient by the time he was thirteen.

At age fourteen, he began getting into trouble. His story is that some other boys shared with him some money they had obtained in a burglary, but Don was picked up by the police. They accused Don of having participated in the crime. Don protested that he was innocent, but the police beat him up unmercifully. That incident, he says, caused him to lose all respect for law and order. When he was sixteen years of age he was expelled from school for fighting. All of his subsequent jobs ended with him getting into arguments with his bosses and quitting or being fired. He became a burglar and was caught several times. By the age of 18, he was in the penitentiary. He was put on hard labor, which he says left him in superb physical condition. Don says that during his life he was arrested approximately 75 times, about 50 being for traffic offenses, 20 for misdemeanors and 2 for felonies.

When Don was 19 years of age he married for the first time. He and his wife stayed together for eight years, having five children. While married, Don worked at several jobs, mostly heavy labor or painting, but he managed to stay out of serious trouble. One day, Don was driving his family home from a picnic. It was raining and he was extremely drunk. His car collided with another which he said was running a stop light, and Don sustained a spinal cord injury. He says that while he was being taken to the hospital, the ambulance crew stopped to have dinner on the way.

Hospital Experiences

Don remembered his hospital experience as one in which all the staff, especially the physicians, were not merely incompetent but seemed to enjoy seeing patients suffer. They filled him up with morphine so that he did not care what they did to him. Then they failed to care for him properly and seemed to be delighted when his bed sores grew big enough to be operated on.

Doctors were not his only enemies. A priest came to see him, but Don did not trust the priest, either. He was pretty sure that the priest was making out with Don's wife on the side.

For quite some time, he was being given heavy doses of Nembutal and codeine, and then one day a doctor abruptly stopped all his medications and Don went into serious withdrawal. A night nurse saved his life by slipping him some Nembutal and a couple of orderlies began bringing him vodka and marijuana to help him out. Finally, a physician gave him a prescription for Demerol which strung him out, but Don felt that it was badly needed.

While he was in the hospital his wife divorced him, but Don did not mind because, as he put it, "I was making a nurse on every shift . . ." He says one physician diagnosed him as having a C-5 lesion, while others said it was a C-7 or C-8. He believed he had too much sensation for the lesion to be very high. He was given a rhizotomy to control his spasms, but despite the unbelievable pain of the surgical procedure it did not work. Don left the hospital against medical advice, feeling he was lucky to escape with his life.

Following this there were more hospitalizations, more surgical procedures and more drugs before the skin sores healed. Bladder infections were responsible for still more surgery and hospitalizations. Finally, Don was sent to a "real" rehabilitation program. He responded well, at least initially. He benefited particularly from physical therapy because he felt it greatly improved his physical condition, and he completed his GED, which he also appreciated. He worked very briefly in a sheltered workshop, putting nuts on bolts for five cents a box, but he could not tolerate that for very long, so he quit. His doctor told him that with his belligerent attitude he probably was not ever going to make it. Don had married a second time, but during his rehabilitation experience he became depressed, started taking drugs again, and his second wife then divorced him.

Through rehabilitation agencies he arranged to go to college. He started taking amphetamines to keep up the pace. He suffered two more bladder infections, went through another marriage and another divorce. In 1970, his until then readily available street supply of amphetamines dried up. Don saw a number of physicians about his pain and muscle spasms. He refused another rhizotomy and finally found a physician who would prescribe Desbutal for him and who was, Don says, amazed at how effectively it worked. In 1972, the law changed and Desbutal became unavailable. More bladder infections followed, yet another marriage, yet another divorce and a failure to set up a business.

The following illustrates Don's attitudes toward his family. While Don was being studied, his youngest son moved in with him.

As Don put it, "He stole my car, tore it up, caused all kinds of trouble. He's gone now, but Don Junior has moved in with me. He's a fuck up, too. He doesn't want to work or anything."

Drug Use History

As may well be supposed, Don's use of drugs of one kind or another began long before his accident. He started using drugs when he was fourteen years of age. He tried a variety of substances besides alcohol, including opiates, barbiturates, cocaine, amphetamines, sedative-hypnotics, marijuana, tranquilizers, and hallucinogens. He started using amphetamines when he was eighteen, but he later adopted amphetamines as his preferred substance, not because they bring him pleasure but in order to control muscle spasms and pain, and to manage recurrent bouts of depression. He was no longer drinking alcohol at the time he was being studied.

In the 1960s, Don would purchase amphetamines in jars of 1,000. The jars contained all kinds of amphetamines: Benzedrine, Dexedrine (both tablets and spansules), Amodex, Bontrils, Dexamyls or Christmas trees, Ritalin, Desoxyn, some whites and oldtime cartwheels, and a lot of speed he did not even know the names of. He used to keep bowls full of them sitting around the house. He tried injecting amphetamine only once, and then he did so intramuscularly rather than intravenously. The effect was so powerful that he realized he could not handle it again. Besides, he had had enough needles in the hospitals. When legislative actions dried up the street supply of amphetamines he resorted to obtaining them by prescription.

Don is gregarious; he always likes to have people around, but he is not a party goer, so he is nearly always alone when he uses drugs. For him it is now strictly a matter of self-medication. Here is how he described his discomfort and his self-directed therapy:

> I get a pain right under my shoulder blade; it's there constantly. If I am out of amphetamines for five to seven days, it will get so bad that nothin', I mean nothin', can kill it. My legs jump some all the time. Speed can cut the spasms at least in half and sometimes as much as 70% after I've been on it two

or three days. You will think this is crazy, maybe, but good grass will sometimes stop the jumping completely. The trouble is that three joints of grass that is good enough to eliminate the spasms will simply knock me on my ass. I can't function on it.

I have told neurologists again and again how it helps me, and they just say, "This guy is a junkie who wants something else."

I have to take biphetamine to make the pain bearable and control the spasms in my legs, but amphetamines get me so hyped up that I can't sleep. Then I have to use barbs or good grass, which is illegal, to sleep. If I take too much of those I get so sluggish I can't function, so I have to take more biphetamines. I have to fight with the doctors to get the amphetamines and break the laws to get the grass.

It is suggestive to note that Malec, Harvey, and Cayner (1982) found that 21 of 24 persons they examined who had experienced the effects of marijuana on spasticity reported a reduction in spasticity associated with marijuana use. Jasinski and Preston (1986) studied how adult males, who were currently non-drug-dependent but who had histories of long-term opiates use, responded to morphine, d-amphetamine and combinations of the two substances. The investigators found that both substances alone were effective but that the combination of the two was even more so. Jasinski and Preston believed that the combination of these substances in therapeutic doses might be useful in treating pain. They also noted, however, that it has a rather high potential for abuse because of the additive euphoria produced by the combined effects of the two drugs.

SOME CONCLUDING THOUGHTS

The research on Don J. was not meant to be a study of rehabilitation process or outcome, nor was it meant to be a study of how to reduce drug use. It illustrates what can be learned by adopting a personological perspective on the problem of chemical substance abuse by persons with disabilities.

The incident that led to Don's disability can be thought of as being one of many manifestations of a lifestyle of defiance, impulsive action, and self-defeating behavior. Don's reaction to his physical condition is at least as much a reaction to his feelings about the authority figures represented by the physicians who have treated him. For Don J., physicians are no more to be trusted than were the police who arrested him and beat him up when he was twelve years old.

Don's story speaks for itself. In one all important respect his life is truly representative. It shows that all aspects of a person's life situation are inextricably intertwined. One cannot speak meaningfully about this man's disability nor about his reaction to it without speaking as well about his drug use. One cannot speak meaningfully about his use of drugs without speaking also about his disability. Neither of these is understandable except in the context of Don's entire life history and current situation.

VALUES

With regard to treatment and rehabilitation, studies like this are almost certain to arouse emotions and stimulate the making of value judgments. Does this man's story arouse your sympathy or your anger? Do you feel that his actions, attitudes and feelings are justified or unjustified? Are you inclined to believe his stories or to think that much of what he told us is no more than a pack of self-serving deceptions? Is there hope for him? Does he deserve help, or do you feel that he has exhausted all reasonable possibilities?

Another set of interesting questions concern Don's hospital and rehabilitation experiences. Was everything done for this man that could have or should have been done? Perhaps some of Don's apparent personal weaknesses, such as his belligerence, could have been interpreted as potential strengths and used in developing a rehabilitation plan that was more suited to his character and that might not have included working in a sheltered workshop. For example, based on his past positive response to hard physical labor and exercise, Don might have enjoyed body building, and he might have benefited from participating in some form of competitive activity. Something else might have been found that would take advantage of his aggressive nature and his fairly high verbal intelligence. Consider how effective he might have become as an advocate for the rights of all persons with disabilities, if he had been helped early on to reexamine his own life and identify with his condition in a constructive rather than a self- destructive way. Perhaps psychological counseling might have helped him do that.

It is well for questions such as these to arise and case study material, particularly that which involves complex and difficult people like Don, nearly always provokes them. Such questions serve as reminders that rehabilitation is not a simple matter of making someone better. To the extent possible, rehabilitation decisions are based on facts, but in the end they are value judgments, whether the professionals who make them want them to be so or not. The close study of individuals provides a means for making values explicit and for exposing to view the bases upon which decisions are made as well as the criteria by which their effectiveness is judged. But even carefully conducted personological research cannot be expected to provide simple answers overnight. What is needed is a systematic approach to the development of a resource base of carefully collected, closely analyzed, and critically evaluated Representative Case Research from which a cumulative body of rehabilitation-relevant knowledge about physical disability and chemical dependence can be extracted. This knowledge can be used to direct rehabilitation care in a manner that is likely to be far more effective and is certain to be more sensitive to the needs of rehabilitation recipients.

REFERENCES

Goldstein, K. (1942). *After-effects of injuries in war*. New York: Grune & Stratton.

Goldstein, K. (1940). *Human nature in the light of psychopathology*. Cambridge, MA: Harvard University Press.

Goldstein, K. (1939). *The organism: a holistic approach to biology derived from pathological data in men*. New York: American Book Co.

Gordon, J., & Shontz, F.C. (1990a). Living with the AIDS virus: A representative case. *Journal of Counseling and Development, 68*, 287-292.

Gordon, J. & Shontz, F.C. (1990b). Representative case research: A way of knowing. *Journal of Counseling and Development, 69*, 67-69.

Heinemann, A.W., & Shontz, F.C. (1984). Adjustment following disability: Representative case studies. *Rehabilitation Counseling Bulletin, 28*, 3-14.

Jasinski, D.R., & Preston, K.L. (1986) Evaluation of mixtures of morphine and d-amphetamine for subjective and physiological effects. *Drug and alcohol dependence, 17*, 1-13.

Korchin, S.J. & Schuldberg, D. (1981). The future of clinical assessment. *American Psychologist, 36*, 1147-1158.

Malec, J., Harvey, R.F., & Cayner, J.J. (1982). Cannabis effects on spasticity in spinal cord injury. *Archives of Physical Medicine and Rehabilitation, 63*, 116-118.

Murray, H.A. (1938). *Explorations in personality: A clinical and experimental study of fifty men of college age.* New York: Oxford University Press.

Shontz, F.C. (1988). Data collection for evaluating treatment outcomes and program effectiveness. In D.J. Lettieri (ed.) *Research strategies in alcoholism treatment assessment,* pp. 69-82. New York: The Haworth Press.

Smuts, J.C. (1926). *Evolution and Holism.* New York: The Macmillan Publishing Co.

Spotts, J.V., & Shontz, F.C. (1980). *Cocaine users: A representative case approach.* New York: Free Press.

Sutker, P.B., & Allain, A.N. (1988). Issues in personality conceptualizations of addictive behaviors. *Journal of Consulting and Clinical Psychology, 56*, 172-182.

PART II:
UNDERSTANDING THE CAUSES,
TYPES, AND PREVALENCE
OF SUBSTANCE ABUSE

Chapter 4

Substance Use Disorders and Persons with Physical Disabilities: Nature, Diagnosis, and Clinical Subtypes

Thomas F. Babor, PhD

INTRODUCTION

This chapter reviews new developments in the study of psychoactive substance use that have implications for the diagnosis and treatment of persons with physical disabilities. It begins with a general model of substance use disorders that takes into account vulnerability factors, exposure to psychoactive substances, mediating variables, the syndrome of dependence, and problems related to substance misuse. Two components of the model, vulnerability and dependence, are given special emphasis. Vulnerability to substance use disorders is discussed in terms of genetic influences and antecedent personality characteristics. Dependence is conceptualized in terms of the syndrome concept recently incorporated into two major diagnostic classification systems (DSM-IIIR and ICD-10). After reviewing the new diagnostic criteria for abuse and dependence, as well as their theoretical underpinnings, the patterning of substance use disorders is discussed in terms of recent theories of alcoholic subtypes. The chapter concludes with consideration of how new developments in dependence theory and empirical subtyping may lead to improvements in the early identification and secondary pre-

The writing of this paper was supported in part by grants from the National Institute on Alcohol Abuse and Alcoholism (AA03510) and the National Institute on Drug Abuse (5R01-DA05592).

vention of substance use disorders in persons with physical disabilities.

A GENERAL MODEL OF SUBSTANCE USE DISORDERS

Recent developments in the conceptualization of substance use disorders are consistent with a theoretical model that considers risk, harmful consequences and dependence as independent but potentially interrelated diagnostic categories. Although alcohol and other psychoactive substances exert profound effects on biological systems and behavior, the consequences of chronic or heavy substance use cannot properly be diagnosed or predicted without taking into account a variety of other factors. To the extent that individual differences in vulnerability (e.g., family history), as well as modifying variables such as duration of use, can be specified, more precise diagnosis of a specific substance-related disorder can be made.

A conceptual scheme is illustrated in Figure 1 to show a set of hypothetical relationships among vulnerability, exposure, modifying factors and consequences. Originally described in an article by Babor, Kranzler, and Lauerman (1987) these relationships are portrayed using examples that pertain primarily to alcohol abuse. Nevertheless, the relevance to the problems of drug dependence will be readily apparent.

In Figure 1 the differential risks of experiencing adverse effects of drinking are divided into two elements, vulnerability and exposure. Vulnerability refers to the physiological, psychological or social characteristics of individuals that make them more or less likely to develop alcohol or drug problems. Longitudinal research and retrospective cohort studies have suggested that the risk of alcohol and other drug problems may be greater among individuals having attention deficit disorder, childhood conduct disorder, and family histories of alcoholism (Hesselbrock et al., 1982). Attention deficit disorder, a type of cognitive dysfunction occurring in early childhood, is characterized by attentional problems, hyperactivity and impulsivity. Researchers (Tarter et al., 1977; Alterman & Tarter, 1986) have found a greater prevalence of this disorder in young male alcoholics. Certain childhood and adolescent personality char-

FIGURE 1. Conceptual framework of risks associated with the consumption of alcohol, portrayed in relation to modifying variables, alcohol dependence and harmful consequences. Proposed ICD-10 diagnostic categories are listed under appropriate sections of the conceptual framework.

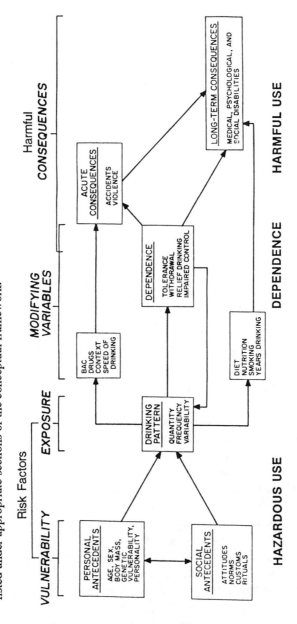

45

acteristics, especially symptoms of shyness, aggression and antisocial behavior, have also been associated with the development of alcohol and other drug problems (Kellam, Ensminger, & Simon, 1980). Familial alcoholism, defined as having an alcoholic first degree relative, has long been considered a predisposing factor for alcoholism. The prevalence of alcoholism in the families of alcoholics is significantly higher than in the families of nonalcoholics, and this association is maintained even when important environmental influences are controlled (Alterman & Tarter, 1986).

Social antecedents may also be considered vulnerability factors. Socially learned attitudes may lead a drinker to expect that alcohol will *cause* the release of aggression or sexual inhibitions, and he or she may act in accordance with these expectations regardless of the pharmacological effects of ethanol. Social norms that encourage daily wine drinking, as in Spain, or which call for severely punishing any alcohol use, as in Islamic societies, may result in drastically different consequences for the substance user. Socially learned drinking customs, like buying rounds or drinking throughout the weekend, may predispose large segments of the male population to drink intensively in response to social pressures. In general, the greater the number of personal and social vulnerability factors, the greater the exposure to drinking or drug use patterns that entail risk. These should be taken into account in the diagnosis of hazardous substance use.

Differential risk is also associated with exposure to alcohol, which to a great extent is influenced by social and economic factors. Since frequent consumption of large amounts of alcohol or other psychoactive substances is a general prerequisite to addiction, those most liable to heavy consumption, such as members of cultural groups which accept high intake, would be at greater risk of developing subsequent problems. Traditionally, emphasis has been placed almost exclusively on the risks associated with exposure to alcohol or other substances over a relatively long period of time. Exposure is in itself complex, entailing such elements as quantity per occasion, frequency of use, and variability of consumption taken over time (Babor, Kranzler, & Lauerman, 1987). The short-term effects of high doses can be as detrimental as chronic use. This kind of exposure increases the risks associated with acute intoxication, such as unintentional injury and overdoses. These risks, however, will be modified by a variety of other factors, depending on how they interact with different aspects of the substance use pattern. The acute consequences of a given dose of ethanol, for example, depend on how fast the beverage is consumed, direction of change in the blood alcohol concentration (BAC) curve, the presence or absence of other drugs in the body, the amount of food the drinker has taken, and the social context of the drinking occasion. Similarly, drug effects are mediated by the mode of administration and the pharmacological properties of the substance.

The long-term consequences of chronic substance use are modified by such lifestyle factors as diet, exercise and the duration of exposure to other harmful substances such as nicotine. In Figure 1, dependence is characterized both by a modifying variable and a risk factor that may intensify substance use. The greater the user's tolerance, for example, the less likely that psychomotor performance will be affected at a given dose. Tolerance, however, may lead to increased consumption, which could increase the risk of chronic disease. Dependence itself can be considered a health consequence to the extent that it disrupts sleep patterns, induces negative mood states, and impairs the user's control over substance ingestion. Within both ICD and DSM, dependence may be diagnosed independent of the harmful consequences of substance use.

NOSOLOGICAL CONCEPTS AND THE SYNDROME CONCEPT OF DEPENDENCE

Classification or nosology is the process of grouping individuals into categories representing specific substance use disorders on the basis of shared characteristics. The precise attributes used to classify a sick person as having a substance use disorder are called diagnostic criteria. The obvious importance of diagnostic criteria derives from their usefulness in making clinical decisions, estimating disease prevalence, and planning treatment.

Alcoholism and drug addiction have been variously defined as medical diseases, mental disorders, behavioral conditions, and in some cases, as the symptom of an underlying mental disorder. The intent of many of these definitions is to permit the classification of alcoholism and drug dependence within standard nomenclatures such as the International Classification of Diseases (ICD) or the Diagnostic and Statistical Manual of Mental Disorders (DSM) of the American Psychiatric Association (World Health Organization, 1989; American Psychiatric Association, 1987).

Recent work on the revision of these two influential diagnostic systems (ICD and DSM) has led to a new concept of dependence, which is now defined as an interrelated syndrome of behavioral, psychological and physical symptoms. Both systems now define dependence according to the elements first proposed by Edwards and Gross (1976). A diagnosis of dependence in the proposed ICD-10 system is made if three or more of the following have been experienced or exhibited at some time in the previous twelve months: (1) a withdrawal state; (2) substance use with the intention of relieving withdrawal; (3) impaired capacity to control the onset, termination or level of use; (4) a narrowing of the personal repertoire of patterns of use, e.g., a tendency to use the substance in the same way on weekdays and weekends, regardless of the social constraints; (5) progressive neglect of alternative pleasures or interests in favor of substance use; and (6) persistence of use despite clear evidence of overtly harmful consequences. DSM-III-R uses a similar set of criteria to diagnose dependence.

A residual category (harmful alcohol use [ICD]; alcohol abuse [DSM]) allows classification of psychological and medical consequences directly related to the ingestion of substances when these are associated with a regular pattern of use. Harmful use is a pattern of using one or more psychoactive substances in a way that causes damage to health. The damage may be (1) physical, such as fatty liver, or accidental injury; or (2) mental (psychological), such as depression or increased depressive episodes related to heavy drinking or drug use. Adverse social consequences that often accompany harmful use, such as employment problems or martial conflict, are not in themselves sufficient to result in a diagnosis of harmful use. They are, however, included within the definition of substance abuse in DSM. This represents an important difference between the two diagnostic systems.

Another concept that was first introduced in a seminal paper on nomenclature and classification (Edwards, Arif, & Hodgson, 1981) is "hazardous use." Hazardous use is a pattern of substance use that will probably lead to harmful consequences for the user. The risk of future damage to health may be physical or mental. This concept is designed to alert health professionals to the potential consequences of more socially acceptable substance use patterns such as social drinking and recreational drug use.

THE SEARCH FOR SUBTYPES

A type is an idealized construction of some observer, based on a combination of biological, psychological or social characteristics, and derived from logical rules that assemble into meaningful clusters individuals who are similar in a majority of relevant respects. Types of alcoholics and drug users have been defined in a variety of ways. Psychoanalytic theorists borrowed from Freud's notions of psychosexual development to characterize alcoholic personality types such as essential and reactive alcoholics. More recently, the application of objective personality tests has led to the development of types based on groupings of abnormal personality traits (Nerviano & Gross, 1983). Another approach to classification has been to generate empirical types by means of cluster analysis, a statistical technique that identifies groups sharing common characteristics. Morey and Skinner (1986), for example, applied cluster analysis to data obtained from an extensive alcohol use questionnaire. Their analysis identified three types of drinkers. Type A (early-stage drinkers) represented a fairly heterogeneous group who showed evidence of drinking problems but had not accrued major symptoms of alcohol dependence. Type B (affiliative, moderate alcohol dependence) drinkers were more socially oriented and tended to drink on a daily basis. Type C (schizoid, severe alcohol dependence) drinkers were more socially isolated, tended to drink in binges, and reported the most severe symptoms of alcoholism. The latter types were found to resemble Jellinek's (1960) delta and gamma species, respectively.

Another approach to the identification of subtypes is based on clinical observation. Zucker's developmental model (1987) is based on the assumption that there are at least four kinds of alcoholism, each having a different developmental process, natural history, and presenting symptoms. Type 1, or antisocial alcoholism, is characterized by the early onset of both antisocial behavior and alcohol-related problems. A genetic influence is suggested by the high prevalence of parental alcoholism and antisocial behavior. This form of alcoholism is generally considered to have a poor prognosis. Type II, termed developmentally cumulative alcoholism, is similar to what other theorists have called primary alcoholism. In this type, the symptomatic drinking behavior is considered to have been established before the onset of any other psychiatric condition. The term developmental cumulative implies that risk is tied to normal, culturally prescribed processes of drinking, rather than childhood antisocial antecedents. Over the course of an individual's drinking career, the addictive process becomes cumulative, assuming a different and more destructive trajectory than if it were simply regulated by normative trends in the culture. Type III, or developmentally limited alcoholism, is characterized primarily by frequent heavy drinking. An extension of adolescent problem drinking, it is often associated with difficulties in separation from the family of origin in young adulthood. This form of problem drinking tends to dissipate in many individuals in the middle twenties with successful assumption of adult career and family roles. Type IV, negative affect alcoholism, tends to be more prevalent in women who use alcohol for affective regulation or to enhance social relationships.

Family history and adoption studies constitute yet another approach to the identification of subtypes. Cloninger (1987) has proposed a neurobiological learning model of alcoholism that distinguishes two basic types, termed "milieu-limited" (Type I) and "male-limited" (Type II). Type I alcoholics tend to have a later onset of alcohol-related problems, develop psychological dependence, and have guilt feelings about their alcohol dependence. In contrast, Type II has an early onset of problems, exhibits spontaneous alcohol-seeking behavior (inability to abstain), and is socially disruptive when drinking. Three dimensions of personality, which in turn have their basis in different neural mechanisms and brain systems, are hypothesized to account for these different types of alcoholism. Thus, Type I is associated with passive-dependent or "anxious" personality traits, while Type II is characterized by traits associated with antisocial personality (i.e., high novelty seeking, low harm avoidance, and low reward dependence). Like Zucker's theory, Cloninger's model implies developmental stages, learning mechanisms, personality variables, and genetic factors in its attempt to account for individual differences in the signs and symptoms of alcoholism.

What is notable about these typological models is that, despite differences in theoretical focus and empirical support, there are some striking similarities in the subtypes they identified. In particular there is sufficient overlap in the characteristics of Zucker's antisocial alcoholic, Cloninger's male-limited type and Morey and Skinner's schizoid drinker to suggest that each theorist is talking about a similar type of alcoholism. This type is characterized by early onset, a more rapid course, more severe symptomatology, greater psychological vulnerability, and poorer prognosis. Another subtype identified by each theorist is the late onset, socially motivated, habitual drinkers variously termed milieu-limited, developmentally cumulative or affiliative alcoholics. This type is characterized by a slower course, fewer complications, less psychological impairment and better prognosis.

IMPLICATIONS FOR UNDERSTANDING SUBSTANCE ABUSE AMONG PERSONS WITH PHYSICAL DISABILITIES

Having outlined some major nosological and diagnostic issues in the conceptualization of substance use disorders, it is now possible to apply these concepts to the explanation of substance abuse among persons with physical disabilities. This will be done by reviewing research related to substance abuse by persons with physical disabilities in relation to the general model outlined in Figure 1.

First, it should be noted that the concepts of hazardous use, harmful use and dependence are best understood within the context of vulnerability, exposure and consequences, as outlined in the model. Hazardous use means that the risks associated with exposure to psychoactive substances are sufficiently great to warrant preventive intervention. Even before a person with a disability begins to experience problems, a high quantity or frequency of substance use should be considered a significant risk factor, particularly when the individual also gives evidence of additional personal or social vulnerabilities. When a high risk pattern of alcohol or drug use is also associated with acute or chronic consequences, then the patient is engaging in harmful use. In the absence of dependence and vulnerability indicators, the course of harmful use can often be benign, with a return of abstinence or social drinking soon after the harmful consequences become apparent. In the case of dependence, the implications are quite different. Not only does dependence increase the likelihood of experiencing both acute and chronic consequences, it also dramatically alters the substance user's chances of controlling substance use. Dependence itself may be related to biological and psychological vulnerabilities. Persons who are prone to personality disorders like sociopathy; who are characterized by shyness, aggressiveness and sensation seeking; and who are born to alcoholic parents, may be prone to a more severe form of dependence than individuals whose dependence develops primarily because of cumulative exposure to ethanol.

Persons with physical impairments are not a homogeneous group, given the broad variety of causes and consequences associated with disability. These include congenital as well as traumatic etiologies; psychological as well as physical impairments; disabilities that affect different organ systems and functional capacities (e.g., visual impairments and seizure disorders); and disease states ranging from chronic degenerative conditions such as arthritis and other rheumatic diseases, to traumatic injuries of the brain and spinal cord. For example, conditions such as gout, an inflammatory reaction manifested by swelling, redness and intense pain in the joints, are sometimes caused by chronic drinking and may in turn exacerbate alcohol consumption, which serves as a temporary relief from chronic pain. Not only do individuals with physical disabilities differ markedly in the nature and severity of their impairment, they also differ with respect to vulnerability factors and exposure to alcohol and other substances.

In a study of drinkers who drive after four or more drinks, Hingson and Howland (1987) found that these individuals are more likely to report speeding, running red lights and driving after smoking marihuana. They are also less likely to use seat belts. These data suggest that there may be greater risk of traumatic injury among heavy drinkers and drug users, especially those who have personality characteristics associated with risk taking and sensation seeking.

O'Donnell et al. (1981-1982), reporting on a survey of 47 patients with spinal cord injury, found that prior to injury many of the patients were physically active, daring individuals who were uninterested in intellectual pursuits. Following injury, restricted mobility was particularly difficult to adapt to, often resulting in misuse of prescription drugs, depression and resumption of drinking and other drug use.

Tarter et al. (1984) found that adolescent sons of alcoholics, who were not themselves alcohol dependent, were more likely than sons of nonalcoholics to have suffered loss of consciousness because of traumatic head injury. Alterman and Tarter (1985) studied the relationship between familial alcoholism and head injury in 76 alcoholic men. Alcoholics with a family history of alcoholism in first degree relatives were more like to have experienced head trauma than nonfamilial alcoholics.

Babor, Kranzler, and Lauerman (1989) interviewed 198 alcoholic and nonalcoholic drinkers to identify vulnerability indicators associated with alcohol abuse. Included in their survey was a scale inquiring about alcohol-related head injury, road crashes and broken bones that occurred since the respondent's eighteenth birthday. Figure 2 shows that when the sample is classified according to their scores on the Michigan Alcoholism Screening Test (Selzer, 1971), there is a strong association in both male and female samples between alcohol problems and alcohol-related trauma. Within the sample of drinkers who were not diagnosed as alcoholic, the study found a strong association between sociopathy and alcohol-related trauma for both males and females. Sociopathy is a general personality trait characterized by strong tendencies to seek stimulation, a diminished capacity to inhibit ongoing behavior, low emotional reactivity, and a diminished capacity to learn from punishing experience.

Moore and Siegal (1989) interviewed 57 college students with orthopedic disabilities about their alcohol and drug use. Among these college students with physical impairments, substance abuse was associated more with a trauma-related disability than with a congenital disability. This was particularly true of students whose injury actually occurred while the individual was under the influence of alcohol or drugs. As in the general college population, a measure of problematic substance use was correlated with thrill-seeking attributes and a previous history of drug use.

These studies suggest that certain vulnerability factors, such as family history, sensation seeking, and sociopathy, thought to influence the patterning and course of substance use disorders, may be prevalent among persons with physical disabilities, particularly those with traumatic injuries that have an onset in adulthood. Given the association of these vulnerabilities with both the early development of substance use disorders and with the manifestation of a more severe course, it would seem particularly important to take these factors into account in diagnosis and treatment planning.

A related aspect of the clinical picture is exposure to alcohol and

FIGURE 2. Trauma scale scores obtained by three drinker groups: (a) patients achieving low MAST scores, (b) patients achieving high MAST scores (in the "alcoholic" range), and (c) diagnosed alcoholics in treatment. Scores are reported separately for males and females.

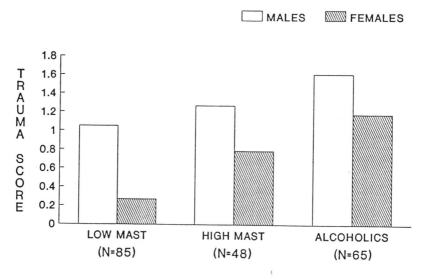

other substances. Although persons with physical disabilities in general may be more likely to abuse alcohol and other drugs than persons without disability (Moore & Siegal, 1989), it is important to consider the patterns of substance use that are associated with particular physical disabilities. Elevated blood alcohol levels have been observed in high proportions of patients encountered in emergency rooms or admitted to hospitals because of traumatic head injury. Exposure to alcohol is a strong predisposing factor in the occurrence of traumatic brain injury (Jones, 1989), spinal cord injury (Heinemann, Donohue, & Schnoll, 1988) and a variety of other physical disabilities, such as gout, arthritis (Nashel, 1989) and seizure disorders (Stoil, 1989).

Following the development of a physical disability, exposure to alcohol and other substances is a prerequisite to the development of substance use disorders. Although persons with physical disabilities may have limited access to alcohol and drugs, a common occurrence is the enlistment of family and friends as suppliers of psychoactive substances. Another source of exposure is prescription medications that are provided for medical and psychological purposes.

The associations among vulnerability, exposure and consequences suggest several possible ways of subtyping persons with disabilities who are using psychoactive substances hazardously or who have begun to experience harmful consequences. Glass (1980-1981), for example, has differentiated between Type A drinkers (those with drinking problems before disability) and Type B drinkers (those with drinking problems after the onset of disability). He suggests that Type A drinkers have less favorable rehabilitation outcomes. Applying this distinction to a sample of 103 patients with spinal cord injuries who were interviewed over an 18-month period, Heinemann, Doll, and Schnoll (1989) found that 65% of the sample were Type A drinkers, 6% were classified as Type B drinkers, and 29% reported no drinking problems either before or after their injuries. Within the category of Type A drinkers, it may be useful to further differentiate those patients who have high degrees of vulnerability and exposure from those who have few vulnerability factors and a low degree of prior exposure to substance use. Evidence from the alcohol literature (Babor & Dolinsky, 1988) suggests that those typological distinctions have important implications for planning treatment and predicting natural history.

In summary, the following generalizations are derived from research that has investigated the relation between substance abuse and physical disability:

1. A majority of individuals with physical impairments and who also have alcohol and other substance-related problems show evidence of such problems prior to onset of impairment.
2. A large proportion of these individuals became physically impaired as a result of trauma and other physical consequences caused directly or indirectly by the use of alcohol or other drugs.
3. A small minority of individuals with physical impairments begin to abuse alcohol and other substances after the onset of impairment.
4. Alcohol and drug abuse may be part of a broader set of personality traits and predispose an individual to both physical disability and substance use disorders.
5. Differential diagnosis of clinical subtypes based on indicators of vulnerability, exposure and consequences may improve treatment planning.

IMPLICATIONS FOR DIAGNOSIS, EARLY IDENTIFICATION, AND TREATMENT MATCHING

In their 18-month follow-up study of patients with spinal cord injuries, Heinemann, Doll, and Schnoll (1989) found that the proportion of drinkers declined following injury. In the six months before injury, 65% of the sample reported one or more drinking problems; the rates were 17% and 24% at six months and 18 months post-injury, respectively. This reduction occurred in the relative absence of professional intervention, as determined by questions about the perceived need for treatment and whether they had actually received treatment.

Given the dramatic social, psychological, and physical readjustments that are required following the onset of physical disability, it is not surprising that substance use would decline during this period. Nevertheless, this spontaneous remission may be deceiving when considered in terms of the long-term prognosis of these patients, many of whom will return to harmful substance use. This raises the possibility that the onset of disability may constitute an important opportunity for external agents to intervene on behalf of substance abusers.

This may be best accomplished by a combination of screening, differential diagnosis, graduated intervention and treatment matching. The process of screening and differential diagnosis should begin with simple self-report screening interviews such as the Alcohol Use Disorders Identification Test (AUDIT) (Babor, de la Fuente, Saunders, & Grant, 1989) and the Drug Abuse Screening Test (DAST) (Skinner, 1982). The AUDIT, reproduced in Table 1, screens for hazardous and harmful alcohol use as well as the presence of dependence symptoms. Such screening should look for signs of substance abuse both before and after the development of physical impairment. For those who screen positive, there is a need to differentiate between patients whose substance use disorder predates their physical disability and those who begin to use psychoactive substances following the onset of disability. More importantly, it is likely that patients with a history of alcoholism in their family, and who exhibit antisocial personality traits, early onset of substance abuse and other types of psychopathology (e.g., anxiety disorder, depression), may be at high risk of resuming their substance abuse following the onset of their disability. Standardized diagnostic interviews are available to collect information about these signs, symptoms and vulnerability factors.

Treatment intervention, especially with individuals who do not have a clear history of chronic alcohol or drug abuse, might best begin with patient education and brief intervention modeled after the brief therapies that have been successful with smokers and heavy drinkers (Babor, Ritson, & Hodgson, 1986). Brief intervention may be all that is necessary for patients who do not give evidence of vulnerability elements. It is also important to provide alcohol and drug education to family members, warning them of the potential hazards of acting as the patient's enabler.

For patients who have developed clear signs of substance abuse

Table 1
The Audit Questionnaire*

1. How often do you have a drink containing alcohol?
   (0) NEVER (1) MONTHLY (2) TWO TO FOUR (3) TWO TO THREE (4) FOUR OR MORE
              OR LESS   TIMES A MONTH   TIMES A WEEK   TIMES A WEEK

2. *How many drinks containing alcohol do you have on a typical day when you
   are drinking? [CODE NUMBER OF STANDARD DRINKS]**
   (0) 1 OR 2 (1) 3 OR 4 (2) 5 OR 6 (3) 7 TO 9 (4) 10 OR MORE.

3. How often do you have six or more drinks on one occasion?
   (0) NEVER (1) LESS THAN (2) MONTHLY   (3) WEEKLY   (4) DAILY OR
                 MONTHLY   ALMOST DAILY

4. How often during the last year have you found that you were not able to
   stop drinking once you had started:
   (0) NEVER (1) LESS THAN (2) MONTHLY   (3) WEEKLY   (4) DAILY OR
                 MONTHLY   ALMOST DAILY

5. How often during the last year have you failed to do what was normally
   expected from you because of drinking?
   (0) NEVER (1) LESS THAN (2) MONTHLY   (3) WEEKLY   (4) DAILY OR
                 MONTHLY   ALMOST DAILY

6. How often during the last year have you needed a first drink in the
   morning to get yourself going after a heavy drinking session?
   (0) NEVER (1) LESS THAN (2) MONTHLY   (3) WEEKLY   (4) DAILY OR
                 MONTHLY   ALMOST DAILY

7. How often during the last year have you had a feeling of guilt or remorse
   after drinking?
   (0) NEVER (1) LESS THAN (2) MONTHLY   (3) WEEKLY   (4) DAILY OR
                 MONTHLY   ALMOST DAILY

8. How often during the last year have you been unable to remember what
   happened the night before because you had been drinking:
   (0) NEVER (1) LESS THAN (2) MONTHLY   (3) WEEKLY   (4) DAILY OR
                 MONTHLY   ALMOST DAILY

9. Have you or someone else been injured as a result of your drinking?
   (0) NO   (2) YES, BUT NOT IN   (4) YES, DURING
                       THE LAST YEAR   THE LAST YEAR

10. Has a relative or friend or a doctor or other health worker, been
    concerned about your drinking or suggested you cut down?
    (0) NO   (2) YES, BUT NOT IN   (4) YES, DURING
                       THE LAST YEAR   THE LAST YEAR

*Numbers in the parentheses are scoring weights. See manual for scoring procedures and interpretation (Babor et al., 1989).

**In determining the response categories it has been assumed that one "drink" contains 10g alcohol. In countries where the alcohol content of a standard drink differs by more than 25% from 10g, the response category should be modified accordingly.

or dependence in the context of a physical disability, more intensive treatment should be considered. Here it is important to differentiate between patients with evidence of early onset, family history, anti-social personality and other vulnerability elements, and those who do not have these antecedents. For the former patients, there is some evidence (Kadden et al., 1989) that structured, cognitive-behavioral, skills training approaches may be more effective than confrontational approaches or those based on interpersonal or psychodynamic therapies. For patients who do not have these vulnerability elements, interpersonal psychotherapies may be more effective.

A major consideration in the effective delivery of all treatment for persons with physical impairments is the degree to which a therapeutic intervention can be tailored to the unique and often daunting circumstances that dominate the daily lives of these individuals.

REFERENCES

Alterman, A.I., and Tarter, R.E. (1986). Hyperactivity and alcoholism: Familial and behavioral correlates. *Addictive Behaviors, 7*, 413-421.

Alterman, A.I., and Tarter, R.E. (1985). Relationship between familial alcoholism and head injury. *Journal of Studies on Alcoholism 46*(3), 256-258.

American Psychiatric Association (1987). *Diagnostic and Statistical Manual of Mental Disorders*, 3rd ed., revised, Washington, DC.

Babor, T.F., and Dolinsky, Z.S. (1988). Alcoholic typologies: Historical evolution and empirical evaluation of some common classification schemes. In R.M. Rose & J.E. Barrett (Eds.), *Alcoholism: Origins and Outcome*, pp. 245-266.

Babor, T.F., Kranzler, H.R., and Lauerman, R.L. (1987). Social drinking as a health and psychosocial risk factor: Anstie's limit revisited. In M. Galanter (Ed.), *Recent Developments in Alcoholism*, Vol. 5. New York: Plenum Press, pp. 373-402.

Babor, T.F., Kranzler, H.R., and Lauerman, R.L. (1989). Early detection of harmful alcohol consumption: Comparison of clinical, laboratory and self-report screening procedures. *Addictive Behaviors, 14*, 139-157.

Babor, T.F., Ritson, E.B., and Hodgson, R.J. (1986). Alcohol-related problems in the primary health care setting: A review of early intervention strategies. *British Journal of Addiction, 81*, 23-46.

Babor, T. F., de la Fuente, J.R., Saunders, J., and Grant, M. (1989). *AUDIT: The Alcohol Use Disorders Identification Test, Guidelines for Use in Primary Health Care*. Geneva, Switzerland: World Health Organization.

Cloninger, C.R. (1987). Neurogenetic adaptive mechanisms in alcoholism. *Science, 236*, 410-416.

Edwards, G., Arif, A. and Hodgson, R. (1981). Nomenclature and classification of drug-and alcohol-related problems: A WHO memorandum. *Bulletin of the World Health Organization, 59,* 225-242.

Edwards, G. & Gross, M.M. (1976). Alcohol dependence: Provisional description of a clinical syndrome. *British Medical Journal, 1,* 1058-1061.

Glass, E. (1980-1981). Problem drinking among the blind and visually impaired. *Alcohol Health and Research World, 5*(2), 20-25.

Heinemann, A.W., Doll, M. & Schnoll, S. (1989). Treatment of alcohol abuse in persons with recent spinal cord injuries. *Alcohol Health and Research World, 13*(2), 110-117.

Heinemann, A.W., Donohue, R. & Schnoll, S. (1988). Alcohol use by persons with recent spinal cord injury. *Archives of Physical Medicine and Rehabilitation, 69,* 619-624.

Hesselbrock, V.M., Stabenau, J.R., Hesselbrock, M.N., Meyer, R.E., & Babor, T.F. (1982). The nature of alcoholism in patients with different family histories for alcoholism. *Prog Neurophyschopharmacol Biol Psychiatry, 6,* 607-614.

Hingson, R., & Howland, J. (1987). Prevention of drunk driving crashes involving young drivers: An overview of legislative countermeasures. In T. Benjamin (Ed.) *Young Drivers Impaired by Alcohol and Drugs.* London: Royal Society of Medicine, pp. 337-348.

Jellinek, E.M. (1960). Alcoholism a genus and some of its species. *Canadian Medical Association Journal, 83,* 1341-1345.

Jones, V.A. (1989). Alcohol abuse and traumatic brain injury. *Alcohol Health and Research World, 13,* 104-109.

Kadden, R.M., Cooney, N. L., Getter, H., & Litt, M.D. (1989). Matching alcoholics to coping skills or interactional therapies: Posttreatment results. *Journal of Consulting and Clinical Psychology, 57*(6), 698-704.

Kellam, S.G., Ensminger, P.E. & Simon, M.D. (1980). Mental health in first grade and teenage drug, alcohol and cigarette use. *Drug and Alcohol Dependence, 5*(4), 273-304.

Moore, D. & Siegal, H. (1989). Double trouble: Alcohol and other drug use among orthopedically impaired college students. *Alcohol Health and Research World, 13*(2), 119-123.

Morey, L.C. & Skinner, H.A. (1986). Empirically derived classifications of alcohol-related problems. In M. Galanter (Ed.), *Recent developments in alcoholism,* vol. V. New York: Plenum Press, pp. 145-168.

Nashel, D.J. (1989). Arthritic disease and alcohol abuse. *Alcohol Health and Research World, 13*(2), 125-127.

Nerviano, V.J. & Gross, H.W. (1983). Personality types of alcoholics on objective inventories. *Journal of Studies on Alcohol, 44,* 837-851.

O'Donnell, J.J., Cooper, J.E., Gessner, J.E., Shehan, I. & Ashley, J. (1981/1982). Alcohol, drugs and spinal cord injury. *Alcohol Health and Research World, 6*(2), 27-29.

Selzer, M.L. (1971). The Michigan Alcoholism Screening Test: The quest for a new diagnostic instrument. *American Journal of Psychiatry, 127,* 1653-1658.

Skinner, H.A. (1982). The drug abuse screening test. *Addictive Behaviors, 7*, 363-371.

Stoil, M.J. (1989). Epilepsy, seizures, and alcohol. *Alcohol Health and Research World, 13*(2), 139-143.

Tarter, R.E., McBride, H., Bounpane, N., & Schneider, D.U. (1977). Differentiation of alcoholics; childhood history of minimal brain dysfunction, family history, and drinking pattern. *Archives of General Psychiatry, 34*, 761-768.

Tarter, R.E., Hegedus, A.M., Goldstein, G., Shelly, C. & Alterman, A.I. (1984). Adolescent sons of alcoholics: Neuropsychological and personality characteristics. *Alcoholism: Clinical and Experimental Research, 8*, 216-222.

World Health Organization, I.C.D. 10. (1989). Draft of Chapter V, *Categories F00- F99, Mental, Behavioral and Developmental Disorders: Clinical Descriptions and Diagnostic Guidelines*. Geneva, Switzerland: World Health Organization.

Zucker, R.A. (1987). The four alcoholisms: A developmental account of the etiologic process. In P.C. Rivers and N.B. Lincoln (Eds.) *Alcohol and Addictive Behavior*. University of Nebraska Press, pp. 27-83.

Chapter 5

Prevalence and Consequences of Alcohol and Other Drug Problems Following Spinal Cord Injury

Allen W. Heinemann, PhD

The prevalence of alcohol-related problems in persons who incur traumatic spinal cord injuries (SCI) and permanent physical disabilities has emerged as a compelling issue in physical medicine and rehabilitation. Alcohol abuse can contribute to onset of disability, impair learning and therefore undermine the rehabilitation process and limit rehabilitation outcomes by contributing to increased morbidity. This is an important issue in light of the great opportunity to prevent post-injury substance abuse and morbidity in persons with SCI who are at risk for post-injury substance abuse. The present chapter describes our knowledge about (1) the prevalence of alcohol and other drug use by persons with SCI, (2) the prevalence of prescription medication misuse in this population, (3) the rate of treatment for substance use problems, (4) the effect of alcohol and other drug use on the rehabilitation process, (5) the effect of alcohol and other drug use on rehabilitation outcome, and (6) the training needs of rehabilitation staff to deal effectively with substance abuse

Support for the research summarized in this chapter was provided by the National Institute on Alcohol Abuse and Alcoholism, National Institute on Disability and Rehabilitation Research, and the Spinal Cord Research Foundation of the Paralyzed Veterans of America.

issues. In doing so, it seeks to provide a base for development of further theory, research, and practice in this area.

PREVALENCE OF ALCOHOL AND OTHER DRUG USE

The prevalence of intoxication at SCI onset has been described by several investigators. O'Donnell, Cooper, Gessner, Shehan, and Ashley (1981-1982) reported a 68% rate of use at spinal cord injury (SCI) onset with 68% resuming drinking during hospitalization. Other studies have found the rate of intoxication for persons incurring traumatic injury to vary between 17% and 49% (Frisbie & Tun, 1984; Fullerton, Harvey, Klein, & Howell, 1981; Galbraith, Murray, Patel, & Knitt-Jones, 1976; Gale, Dikmen, Wyler, Temkin, & McClean, 1983; Heinemann, Goranson, Ginsburg, & Schnoll, 1989). Impaired judgment resulting from intoxication appears to be responsible for increased risk-taking that results in many injuries. The prevalence of alcohol use and abuse following initial care for traumatic disability has been reported in several recent studies. The rate of moderate and heavy drinking reported by vocational rehabilitation and independent living center clients with SCI was nearly twice the rate reported in the general population (46% vs. 25%; Johnson, 1985), while the rate of alcoholic symptomatology has been observed to vary from 49% of persons with recent onset SCI (Heinemann, Donohue, Keen, & Schnoll, 1988) to 62% of vocational rehabilitation facility clients (Rasmussen & DeBoer, 1980). Age-related differences in drinking problems were highlighted in a study of primarily older veterans with SCI (Kirubakaran, Kumar, Powell, Tyler, & Armatas, 1986) whose alcohol and drug use was less than the rate reported in the National Institute on Drug Abuse's National Household Survey (NIDA, 1988). These findings suggest that age-related differences in the rate of alcohol and other drug abuse in the able-bodied population also exist in persons with SCI.

The prevalence of intoxication at time of SCI was examined in 88 cases at admission to our acute SCI center (Heinemann, Schnoll, Brandt, Maltz, & Keen, 1988). Urine and blood samples were obtained from these patients at admission to an acute SCI trauma center. These patients were later admitted consecutively to the Rehabilitation Institute of Chicago. Forty-seven of these individuals also agreed to participate in an ongoing study of drug use and provided information regarding their perception of intoxication at SCI onset. The sample ranged in age from 14 to 60 years ($x = 29.4$ years, SD = 10.8). Men composed 85% of the sample. The majority of the sample was white (67%); the most frequent cause of injury was road and traffic accidents (44%); quadriplegia was the resulting disability for 70% of the sample. Participant and nonparticipant groups did not differ in terms of age, gender, race, injury etiology, nor disability. Also, the groups did not differ with respect to the incidence of positive urine and serum analysis for 30 substances with abuse potential.

Serum ethanol greater than 50 mg/dl was the most frequently found substance (observed in 40% of the cases) followed by urine analysis evidence of cocaine (14%), cannabinoids (8%), benzodiazipines (5%), and opiates (4%). Evidence of substances with abuse potential was found in urine for 35% of the sample. A total of 62% of the sample had either serum ethanol greater than 50 mg/dl or a positive urine analysis. Care must be taken in interpreting these results as *prima facie* evidence of chemical dependence since false positive results may reflect occasional or low dose use of substances with abuse potential which was detected by toxicology screens.

In the same study at the Rehabilitation Institute of Chicago, substance use histories were obtained from 103 persons with recent SCI (Heinemann, Donohue, Keen, & Schnoll, 1988). The sample consisted of persons, aged 13 to 65 years at injury, who were cognitively intact, injured within the past year, and English speaking. The mean age of the sample was 28.2 years at recruitment; 75% were men. In general, lifetime exposure to and recent use of several substances with abuse potential were greater than for a like-age national sample. Compared with a national sample (National Institute on Drug Abuse, 1988), the SCI sample of 18-25 year olds reported significantly greater (at least 10 percentage points greater) exposure to amphetamines, marijuana, cocaine and hallucinogens. In addition to these four substance categories, the SCI group which was 26 years of age and older reported significantly greater exposure to narcotic analgesics and tranquilizers than did the national sample. Reports of recent substance use in the SCI sample were significantly greater than for the national sample for alcohol, amphetamines, marijuana, cocaine and hallucinogens for the 18-25 year olds. For the SCI group which was 26 years of age and older, recent use was at least 10 percentage points greater than the national sample for tobacco, alcohol, amphetamines and marijuana. Finally, greater proportions of the SCI sample for both the 18 to 25 years and 26 year and older groups reported greater recent use for 9 of 10 substance categories compared to the national sample.

Within the SCI sample, young adults (18 to 25 year olds) reported greater recent use of marijuana and greater cocaine exposure than did the 26 years of age and older group; in contrast, greater tobacco exposure was reported in the 26 years of age and older group. Exposure to tobacco, amphetamines, marijuana, hallucinogens, tranquilizers and sedatives, and recent use of tobacco, alcohol, amphetamines, cocaine and hallucinogens were greater for the 39% who reported being intoxicated at time of injury.

On first inspection, these results suggest that persons incurring SCI are more likely to use and abuse alcohol and other drugs to a greater degree than do persons in the general population. However, before classifying persons that incur SCI as being abuse prone and increasing their stigma further, several methodological considerations must be considered when interpreting these comparisons. Although the methodologies in our study and the National Household Survey were essentially the same, different definitions of recent use require caution against overgeneralizing the results. For instance, recent use criteria of one or more times during the past month vs. three or more times during the past six months may not be assessing substance use in a comparable manner. Despite the complication in interpreting the results, we chose this definition because we sought to exclude occasional or sporadic use. The net effect of these differences may be to minimize rather than to inflate differences, though we did not test this effect.

These results suggest that intoxication at SCI onset is a marker of pre-injury substance use, and that it is important to screen for substance abuse in persons who incur traumatic injury. Implications for clinical practice are apparent since the lifetime exposure to and recent use of substances reported by this sample may place persons with SCI at risk for substance abuse. Many studies have reported a relationship between previous substance use and subsequent use of other drugs (cf., Dembo, Blount, Schmeidler, & Burgos, 1985). While substance use is not necessarily abuse nor does it necessarily result in specific problems, it is important to understand the context, expectancies, and motives for use. For example, substance use may reflect adolescent experimentation, a means of enhancing social interactions, or a pattern of self-destructive behavior. Clinicians should take note of substance use and observe if it signals other problems. Additionally, use of substances with abuse potential may result in a greater likelihood of incurring traumatic injury. Indeed, 39% of the sample stated they were intoxicated at injury onset. Intoxication results in impaired judgment and increases the likelihood of taking risks which may result in physical injury. These results highlight the importance of assessing alcohol and drug abuse related problems so that a potential dual disability is identified and treated in a timely fashion.

PREVALENCE OF PRESCRIPTION MEDICATION MISUSE

In a separate sample of 96 persons with long-term SCI, we examined the use of prescription medication, alcohol and illicit substances and problems resulting from their use as well as depression and disability acceptance. Selection criteria for the sample age was between 13 and 65 years at injury, cognitively intact, injury sustained more than one year earlier, and English speaking. The sample was recruited from members of the Illinois Chapter of the National Spinal Cord Injury Association (NSCIA) and Access Living of Metropolitan Chicago. NSCIA provides organized social, advocacy and public policy programs that appeal to a wide range of persons. While the organization is not representative of all persons with injuries since interest in a special interest group is a prerequisite to participation, membership is open to anyone and the organization has an active outreach program to persons with recent injuries. In contrast, Access Living is an independent living center, and provides housing, transportation and personal care attendant referral to persons with a variety of disabling conditions, including spinal cord injury. While membership in the two organizations overlaps to a small extent, these organizations are unique in being visible and accessible to a wide spectrum of persons with disabilities.

Participants were asked if they had ever used substances in each of 15 categories, and if so, whether they had used substances in each of these categories on three or more occasions during the past six months. The prescription categories included diazepam, sedatives and hypnotics, barbiturates, aspirin or acetaminophen with codeine, propoxyphene, antidepressants, anticholinergics, amphetamines, and narcotic analgesics. Participants using prescription medications were asked if the drug was prescribed and if they used it as prescribed; prescription misuse was defined as use of a prescribed medication more often or in greater quantity than was prescribed, or using these medications without a prescription. Nonprescription substances included alcohol, marijuana, cocaine, psychedelics, phencyclidine, and inhalants. Finally, participants were asked if they experienced one or more problems resulting from their use of each substance category; potential problems included loss of control over amount used; disruptions with family and friends; cognitive, affective, health, sexual, financial, driving and employment problems; fatigue; and agitation. Linkowski's (1971) Acceptance of Disability Scale and Beck's Depression Inventory (1967) were also completed by participants.

The mean age of the sample was 38.5 years; SCI occurred an average of 12.6 years earlier; 70% were men; 57% were quadriplegic; and 59% were employed. Forty-three percent of the sample used prescription medications with abuse potential, and of these persons, 24% reported misusing one or more medications on one or more occasions. Persons who regularly used prescription medications were less accepting of their disability and were more depressed than were persons who were not using prescription medications. Additionally, persons reporting problems resulting from prescription medication use were more depressed, and persons reporting problems resulting from nonprescription substance use were less accepting of their disability than were persons not reporting these problems.

Unexpectedly, misuse of prescription medication occurred independent of nonprescription substance use; persons who used prescription medications were no more or less likely to use nonprescription substances than were nonusers of prescription medications. Prescription misuse appears to be a different phenomenon than nonprescription substance abuse. Interestingly, prescription misuse, *per se*, was not associated with poorer psychological adjustment. While the rate of prescription misuse was not greater in this sample compared to the general adult population, the kinds of drugs which were misused did differ. Diazepam and propoxyphene were most often misused in this sample, while stimulants are most often misused by the general adult population.

These results suggest that use of prescription and nonprescription substances by persons with SCI is associated with negative psychological outcomes and that prescription misuse should be monitored as a potential complication. Clinicians should attend to depression and poor psychological adjustment which may underlie medical complications. Training physicians, nursing and allied health staff to recognize prescription medication misuse and to understand the reasons for misuse emerges as an important task in enhancing the rehabilitation outcomes.

RATE OF TREATMENT FOR SUBSTANCE USE PROBLEMS

We also studied the rate of self-reported substance use, consequent problems, perceived need for treatment, and receipt of treatment by persons with long-term SCI (Heinemann, Doll, Armstrong, Schnoll, & Yarkony, 1991). Participants were interviewed on four occasions that covered the six-month time period before injury, injury to one year before first interview (which averaged 13 years), the year before the first interview and a subsequent one year period. A total of 86 persons with traumatic SCI participated; they ranged from 13 to 58 years of age at injury, and were interviewed an average of 13 years later. The categories of substances and potential problems resulting from use were the same as described above.

All participants reported use of substances with abuse potential on three or more occasions at one or more of these time periods; the time of greatest use was injury to six months before first interview; the duration of this period ranged from 18 months to 43 years.

Problems resulting from substance use were reported by 70% during one or more of the assessment periods. However, only 16% reported perceiving a need for treatment of substance abuse and 7% actually received treatment. Reasons given for not seeking treatment included believing that they could change their substance use without treatment (reported by 28% of the untreated participants), changing their minds about the need for treatment (12%), believing that they could not change their use (8%), being unable to afford treatment (3%), and saying that treatment was not necessary (3%). While the incidence of self-recognized substance use problems may be low, the total number of persons may be substantial.

The number of substance use problems averaged 2.1 for the 33 persons reporting problems before injury, 1.9 for 45 persons reporting problems during the period from injury to one year before the first interview, 1.8 for 25 persons reporting problems during the year before the first interview, and 1.5 for 23 persons reporting problems during the year before the second interview. The number of problems experienced at each time period were positively correlated with the number of substance use problems during preceding time periods, indicating that persons experiencing more problems at earlier periods were more likely to report problems at the next period.

These results demonstrate that spinal cord injury does no more to cure substance abuse for some persons than does other life disruptions such as job loss, divorce, and other forms of trauma. These results do help inform us about stages of change in addiction processes and highlight that use patterns may vary from substance to substance and with time. For treatment to be successful, we need to understand the context in which substance use problems develop, to recognize problems when they occur, and to develop means to control or end substance abuse. Timely assessment of substance abuse and provision of treatment services to persons with traumatic injury is indicated to prevent a potential dual disability.

EFFECTS OF ALCOHOL AND OTHER DRUG USE ON REHABILITATION PROCESS

In addition to reporting pre-disability alcohol use, the Rehabilitation Institute of Chicago patient sample with recent injuries also described their activity patterns during their inpatient rehabilitation stay (Heinemann, Goranson, Ginsburg, & Schnoll, 1989). They described their activities in a structured interview format using the Activity Pattern Indicators (API) (Diller, Fordyce, Jacobs, & Brown, 1981). The API is a functional status assessment measure of time spent in several classes of activity (vocational, educational, rehabilitation, sleep, personal care, family role, TV watching, social activity, and travel). It is completed in an interview format with a trained research assistant. Persons indicate activity performed, beginning and ending times, where the activity occurred, who else was present, whether the activity was supervised or whether any physical assistance was received, and whether any other activity occurred concurrently. A weekday and weekend day were assessed at each evaluation period. Activities were summed into four categories: productive activities such as rehabilitation, quiet time such as sleeping, social activities, and quiet recreation.

The frequency and quantity of alcohol use was recorded separately for weekdays and weekends during the six months before injury. These variables were factor analyzed because they were highly correlated; a single factor accounting for 73% of the variance in these variables was extracted. Drinking problems were assessed as described above.

A family history of alcoholism was reported by 29% of the sample. Persons who reported drinking more often and whose drinking resulted in problems before injury were more likely to be drinking when injury occurred, regardless of age, gender, or family history of alcoholism. As expected, pre-disability drinking and family history of drinking problems were related to the number of drinking problems reported. Path analysis was used to examine a hypothesized model in which specific variables (e.g., family drinking problems, drinking problems, level of injury) were used to predict outcomes (disability acceptance, activity patterns). Persons who drank more before injury and who reported more family drinking problems also reported a greater number of drinking problems; in turn, persons with more drinking problems reported spending less time in quiet activities such as sleeping and resting during rehabilitation hospitalization, but spent more time in quiet recreation (e.g., watching television and reading). Furthermore, persons who drank more before injury reported spending less time in productive activities such as rehabilitation therapies.

The finding that heavier preinjury drinkers spent less time in rehabilitation activities is disturbing since these activities provide the information and experiences which help make the transition from hospital to home more successful. It may be that persons who drink often and heavily experience drinking-related problems; in turn, they spend time and energy coping with these drinking-related problems rather than participating in activities which prepare them for life in their communities. While these relationships need to be studied over time to determine if and how long they persist, they do highlight important factors which may affect rehabilitation outcome.

EFFECTS OF ALCOHOL AND OTHER DRUG USE ON REHABILITATION OUTCOME

Substance use is a concern for young adults because peak use often occurs when they are making critical commitments to social and vocational roles. Impaired performance as a student, worker, or family member can have lifelong effects. More immediate effects are also apparent as unemployment is consistently associated with high frequency substance use, particularly alcohol and illegal substances other than marijuana (Brunswick, 1979). Consequently, we examined the relationship between changes in employment status, substance use, depression and disability acceptance following SCI in the sample of community residents. Participants completed the Beck Depression Inventory and Linkowski's Acceptance of Disability Scale. Using Hollingshead and Redlich's Social Position Index to code social status, 21% were employed at the same status as before injury, 16% were employed and had increased job status, 23% became employed, 18% became unemployed and 22% remained unemployed. Employed individuals were less likely to use diazepam (Valium), alcohol, marijuana and cocaine. Persons who were unemployed at injury onset and became employed and persons who increased in SPI score between injury and interview reported greater disability acceptance. Further, persons who used prescription drugs in either a prescribed or nonprescribed manner were more depressed and less accepting of their disability than were persons who used no prescription drugs.

While the finding of an association between substance use and employment does not allow us to determine which is cause and effect, the relationship between these variables should alert us to the critical role of substance use after injury and encourage clinicians to explore the meaning it has in the lives of users. Clearly, vocational rehabilitation outcomes can be impaired by substance use. This remains as an issue to be addressed by rehabilitation professionals.

TRAINING NEEDS OF REHABILITATION STAFF

Rehabilitation staff training emerges as an important need given the rate of substance abuse in this population. Physicians', nurses' and allied health team members' ability to detect, evaluate, and intervene with patients who abuse alcohol or other drugs is critical in providing comprehensive clinical care. We assessed rehabilitation medicine residents' training, knowledge about, and attitudes toward chemical dependence in a nationwide survey (Shade-Zeldow, Roth, Heinemann, Kiley, Doll, & Yarkony, 1990). Of 76 residency programs, directors of 49 (64%) agreed to distribute surveys to residents. A total of 335 forms were returned. A 46-item questionnaire was developed to assess substance abuse related information. The number of correct responses was unrelated to hours of instruction in substance abuse, but was related to extent of comfort addressing alcohol and other drug problems. Greater knowledge about substance abuse issues may allow clinicians to address patient needs more comfortably and frequently.

A similar survey was conducted with members of the American Congress of Rehabilitation Medicine, a professional organization with physician, nursing, and allied health members (Kiley, Heinemann, Shade-Zeldow, Doll, Roth, & Yarkony, 1992). A total of 3,305 members were mailed the questionnaire; a 37% response rate was obtained with two follow-up letters to nonrespondents. Respondents included physicians (61% of the total), nursing and allied health clinicians (25%) and other members (14%). Respondents reported a mean of 12 years experience in rehabilitation and an average of 62% of time spent in patient care activities. Members suspected that 29% of their patients with traumatic injuries had alcohol or drug abuse problems. Routine screening for alcohol and other drug problems at their facility was reported by 30%. Substance abuse education for staff was reported by 50%; patient education regarding substance abuse was reported by 59%. While 79% reported that their facilities had referral procedures for substance abuse problems, only 44% reported making referrals. Members stated that patients were referred most often to Alcoholics Anonymous. Members were optimistic about treatment outcomes for chemical dependence and believed that patients' substance use problems should be addressed concurrently during rehabilitation.

Rehabilitation Institute of Chicago staff developed a substance abuse education program for team members working with patients in spinal cord injury rehabilitation in an effort to enhance the effectiveness of patient care (Heinemann, Kiley, Shade-Zeldow, Roth, & Doll, 1990). The program described a theoretical context within which staff could understand substance use problems, described abusable drugs, reviewed the epidemiology of alcohol and other drug abuse, presented the basic sciences and physiology of alcohol use, described the nature of attitudes toward chemical use, reviewed hospital policies and procedures, and described assessment and referral procedures. The hour-long program was supplemented with printed materials. The effectiveness of the education program was evaluated with a 33-item questionnaire which was administered before and six months after the presentation to assess changes in staff knowledge, attitudes, and behavior. The number of correct responses six months after education was greater for both attendees and nonattendees than at the pre-test. However, improvement in knowledge was greater for staff who attended the education program than for staff who did not attend. Staff who attended the presentation reported making more referrals before and six months after the program than did those who did not attend ($p < .05$). Staff who made the most referrals after education were those who made more referrals before education, who suspected more patients of pre-injury substance abuse, and who had less experience in rehabilitation. The education program did not have a measured effect on attitudes towards substance use. It may have been that the attitude questions did not tap central beliefs, the program was too short, the opportunity for discussion of personal beliefs and concerns too limited, or that other unmeasured factors limited attitude change. Nevertheless, staff consistently expressed attitudes that acknowledged the extent of substance abuse problems faced by patients, were optimistic about chemical dependence treatment efficacy, and were supportive of efforts to help patients deal with chemical dependence issues. They strongly supported a concurrent focus on rehabilitation and substance abuse issues.

The results of these surveys and training experience suggest the need for education regarding substance abuse treatment, facility policies, and referral procedures. The focus of this education should be on early assessment of pre- and post-disability alcohol use and related problems; this training could also help identify persons who are at risk for not availing themselves fully of the rehabilitation services offered during hospitalization. These services may be crucial in promoting adaptation after discharge. Training on interventions designed to increase therapy attendance may be useful, especially if a relationship between the amount of time spent in therapies and future adaptation is found. Assignment of specific responsibilities for assessment of pre-injury alcohol use and related problems is an important prerequisite so that this information is available in planning a rehabilitation program that will benefit persons with heavy drinking or drug using histories. Training on how, when, and to whom to make substance abuse referrals for alcohol treatment should also be provided.

Specific suggestions for enhancing the rehabilitation care and life adaptation of persons with recent SCI are summarized as follows. First, assessment of alcohol use and alcoholism should be a routine part of all inpatient screenings in acute care and rehabilitation programs for persons incurring traumatic injury. Responsibility for this screening could be assumed by a variety of team members including representatives from medicine, nursing, psychology, or social work. Second, training of medical and allied health team members to recognize alcohol abuse is important to allow them to provide this assessment. Alcoholism treatment program professionals could consult with physical medicine and rehabilitation care providers to acquire this knowledge. Third, establishing referral networks to alcohol treatment programs is necessary if a potential dual disability is to be identified and treated in a timely fashion. Sound communication links must be established so that alcohol treatment programs and alcohol counselors learn about the special needs of patients with disabilities. Accessibility needs, functional abilities and attitudes toward persons with disabling conditions are some of the topics that should be addressed in training programs for alcoholism and drug abuse treatment personnel. Chemical dependence treatment programs designed specifically for persons with physical disabilities are another treatment alternative (Anderson, 1980-1981; Krause, 1992; Lowenthal & Anderson, 1980-1981; Sweeney & Foote, 1982), though few are in existence to date.

Finally, hospital policy issues emerge from the findings of this study. Policies regarding possession and use of alcohol as well as recreational or socialization programs that incorporate alcohol use need to be clearly formulated in light of studies examining controlled drinking outcomes. While alcohol used in moderation is likely to pose few problems for many patients, those who have histories of alcohol abuse could be encouraged to abuse alcohol by policies and programs that provide opportunities for alcohol consumption. A case by case assessment of each patient's history and social needs is advised.

To summarize, substance use is often overlooked in rehabilitation settings. Staff who do not know how to recognize substance abuse problems are unlikely to intervene in a timely and effective manner. Referral links to chemical dependence programs are needed if a potential dual disability is to be prevented. Since few speciality programs exist for persons with physical disabilities, rehabilitation staff at facilities across the country should develop links with local programs or develop their own programs, and encourage communication about needs of persons with both physical disabilities and chemical dependence problems.

Early identification of persons with spinal cord injuries who abuse or are addicted to substances should minimize the incidence of secondary complications of SCI, decrease the cost of rehabilitation and improve rehabilitation outcome. Since the annual medical costs for all persons with spinal cord injury is estimated to be greater than $1.9 billion, timely and effective intervention for those persons who abuse or are at risk for chemical abuse is both humane and cost effective.

REFERENCES

Anderson, P. (1980-1981). Alcoholism and the spinal cord disabled: A model program. *Alcohol Health and Research World*, *5*, 37-41.

Beck, A. (1967). *Depression: Causes and Treatment*. Philadelphia: University of Pennsylvania Press.

Brunswick, A.F. (1979). Black youth and drug use behavior. In G. Beschner & A. Friedman (Eds.), *Youth Drug Abuse: Problems, Issues and Treatment* (pp. 443-492). Lexington, MA: Lexington Books.

Dembo, R., Blount, W., Schmeidler, J., & Burgos, W. (1985).Methodological and substantive issues involved in using the concept of risk in research into the etiology of drug use among adolescents. *Journal of Drug Issues*, *15*, 537-553.

Diller, L., Fordyce, W., Jacobs, D. & Brown, M. (1981). *Activity Pattern Indicators Timeline Training Materials*. New York: New York University Medical Center.

Frisbie, J.H. & Tun, C.G. (1984). Drinking and spinal cord injury. *Journal of the American Paraplegia Society*, *7*, 71-73.

Fullerton, D.T., Harvey, R.F., Klein, M.H., & Howell, T. (1981). Psychiatric disorders in patients with spinal cord injuries. *Archives of General Psychiatry*, *38*, 1369-1371.

Galbraith, S., Murray, W.R., Patel, A.R. & Knitt-Jones, R. (1976). The relationship between alcohol and head injury and its effects on the conscious level. *British Journal of Surgery*, *63*, 128-130.

Gale, J.L., Dikmen, S., Wyler, A., Temkin, N. & McClean, A. (1983). Head injury in the Pacific Northwest. *Neurosurgery*, *12*, 487-491.

Heinemann, A., Donohue, R., Keen, M., & Schnoll, S. (1988). Alcohol use by persons with recent spinal cord injuries. *Archives of Physical Medicine and Rehabilitation*, *69*, 619-624.

Heinemann, A., Goranson, N., Ginsburg, K., & Schnoll, S. (1989). Alcohol use and activity patterns following spinal cord injury. *Rehabilitation Psychology*, *34*, 191-206.

Heinemann, A., Doll, M., Armstrong, M., Schnoll, S. & Yarkony, G. (1991). Substance use and receipt of treatment by persons with long-term spinal cord injuries. *Archives of Physical Medicine and Rehabilitation*, *72*, 482-487.

Heinemann, A., Kiley, D., Shade-Zeldow, Y., Roth, E., & Doll, M. (1990). Chemical dependence education for rehabilitation professionals. Paper presented at the annual meeting of the American Congress of Rehabilitation Medicine and the American Academy of Physical Medicine and Rehabilitation, Phoenix, Arizona, 1990.

Heinemann, A., Schnoll, S., Brandt, M., Maltz, R. & Keen, M. (1988). Toxicology screening in acute spinal cord injury. *Alcoholism: Clinical and Experimental Research, 12*, 815-819.

Hollingshead, A., & Redlich, F. (1958). *Social class and mental illness.* New York: John Wiley and Sons.

Johnson, D.C. (1985). Alcohol use by persons with disabilities. Wisconsin Department of Health and Social Services.

Kiley, D., Heinemann, A., Shade-Zeldow, Y., Doll, M., Roth, E. & Yarkony, G. (1992). Rehabilitation professionals' knowledge and attitudes about substance abuse issues. *Journal of NeuroRehabilitation, 2*, 35-44.

Kirubakaran, V.R., Kumar, V.N., Powell, B.J., Tyler, A.J. & Armatas, P. J. (1986.) Survey of alcohol and drug misuse in spinal cord injured veterans. *Journal of Studies on Alcohol, 47*, 223-227.

Krause, J. (1992). Delivery of substance abuse services during spinal cord injury rehabilitation. *Journal of NeuroRehabilitation, 2*, 45-51.

Linkowski, D. (1971). A scale to measure acceptance of disability. *Rehabilitation Counseling Bulletin, 4*, 236-244.

Lowenthal, A. & Anderson, P. (1980-1981). Network development: Linking the disabled community to alcoholism and drug abuse programs. *Alcohol Health and Research World, 5*, 16-19.

National Institute on Drug Abuse (1988). *National Household Survey on Drug Abuse: Main Findings.* Rockville MD: National Institute on Drug Abuse.

O'Donnell, J.J., Cooper, J.E., Gessner, J.E., Shehan, I., & Ashley, J. (1981-1982). Alcohol, drugs and spinal cord injury. *Alcohol Health & Research World, 6*, 27- 29.

Rasmussen, G.A. & DeBoer, R.P. (1980). Alcohol and drug use among clients at a residential vocational rehabilitation facility, *Alcohol Health and Research World, 5*, 48-56.

Shade-Zeldow, Y., Roth, E., Heinemann, A., Kiley, D., Doll, M. & Yarkony, G. (1990). Rehabilitation medicine residents' knowledge regarding substance abuse. Paper presented at the annual meeting of the American Congress of Rehabilitation Medicine and the American Academy of Physical Medicine and Rehabilitation, Phoenix, Arizona, 1990.

Sweeney, T.T. & Foote, J.E. (1982). Treatment of drug and alcohol abuse in spinal cord injury veterans. *International Journal of the Addictions, 17*, 897- 904.

Chapter 6

Prescription Medication in Rehabilitation

Sidney Schnoll, MD, PhD

Patients with disabilities often experience problems that require the use of medications. Those with severe disabilities resulting from spinal cord injuries, traumatic amputations and traumatic brain injuries frequently contract their disability during a period of intoxication with alcohol or other drugs. Although intoxication alone is not sufficient evidence to define someone as an addict, the patient who was intoxicated at the time of injury may be at high risk for abuse of prescribed medications.

Pain syndromes, muscle spasms and sleep problems are treated with narcotic analgesics and sedative-hypnotics: two classes of drugs that have abuse potential. Despite this potential for abuse, patients who need these medications should not be denied them but should be medicated appropriately and monitored carefully to deal with abuse should it occur. This chapter will address the issues regarding the appropriate use of these medications and how to monitor and deal with abuse should it occur.

ADDICTION AND DEPENDENCE

The current diagnostic criteria for dependence on alcohol and other drugs as described in the Diagnostic and Statistical Manual (Third Edition, Revised, 1987) published by the American Psychiatric Association are helpful in diagnosing the chemically dependent person, but they do not differentiate between the patient who has become dependent on prescribed medication but is not abusing it and the patient who abuses the prescribed medication. Because of this problem, the following definitions for addiction and dependence will be used in the context of this chapter.

Dependence: An adaptation of cells in the body to the presence of a drug to the point that when the drug is removed a rebound effect occurs that is called withdrawal. Dependence is a pharmacologic phenomenon. Physicians make people drug dependent quite frequently. A patient who is prescribed narcotics post-operatively becomes dependent. When the patient is taken off the narcotics he or she experiences some withdrawal. If the patient does not develop "drug seeking behavior" the patient is not addicted to the drug. There is growing evidence (Miller & Jick, 1978; Porter & Jick, 1980) that very few patients who are dependent on legitimately prescribed narcotics become addicted. There is similar evidence for low levels of addiction in patients prescribed benzodiazepines for medical reasons (Woods, Katz, & Winger, 1988).

Addiction: A chronic disorder characterized by compulsive use of substances resulting in detrimental psychological, physical, and social consequences and continued use despite evidence of that harm. Addiction is a behavior, a behavior that we do not understand very well, but is clearly different from dependence. Although the two are often closely related and frequently coexist in the same person, they can exist independently.

Another way of explaining the difference between addiction and dependence is that dependence is caused by the pharmacologic properties of the drug and addiction results from some predisposition in the person. The drug may be a catalyst for the development of the behavior but does not cause the behavior in everyone exposed to the drug. Since the drugs do not cause addiction, it is important to know who is at risk for the development of addictive behaviors. It is the patient about whom we are concerned, not the drug. Patient characteristics that place them at high risk for addiction include: (1) a previous history of addiction and/or problem drug use; (2) a family history of addiction in parents, grandparents, aunts, uncles and siblings; and (3) a history of personality disorder, particularly antisocial personality (Goodwin & Warnock, 1991; Cloninger, Bohman, Sigvardsson, 1981; Cloninger, 1987; Miller, Gold, Belkin, Klahr, 1989).

PRESCRIBED DRUGS WITH ABUSE LIABILITY

The two categories of drugs that we are most concerned about as having high abuse potential are the narcotic analgesics (Table 1) and the sedative-hypnotics (Table 2). The narcotic analgesics can be classified into several subcategories: those that are opium derivatives such as morphine and codeine; the semisynthetics, hydromorphone, diacetylmorphine, oxycodone; and the purely synthetic compounds, such as methadone, meperidine and propoxyphene. Another way of categorizing opioids is by their action at the opioid receptors. Drugs that only produce analgesia and other typical effects of morphine are called narcotic agonists. Drugs that block the effects of morphine are called narcotic antagonists. Recently, drugs have been developed that have both agonist and antagonist properties. These drugs are called mixed agonist-antagonist drugs or partial agonists. In low doses they most often act as agonists and as the dose is increased sometimes act more like antagonists, thus reducing the likelihood of overdose and possibly abuse. Partial or mixed agonist drugs include pentazocine, butorphanol, buprenorphine and nalbuphine. Drugs in the mixed or partial agonist group have lower abuse potential than the pure agonists, but they do have potential for abuse as demonstrated by the epidemic of Ts and blues (Talwin and pyribenzamine) abuse that occurred several years ago. Partial agonist drugs have different receptor binding characteristics than the pure agonists. The pure agonists most often bind to the mu receptor and the partial agonists bind to the kappa receptor which produces more dysphoria. This may be an important factor in their reduced abuse potential.

The other important group of drugs is the sedative-hypnotics which include the benzodiazepines, barbiturates, sleeping pills, muscle relaxants and alcohol. The sedative-hypnotics are among the most prescribed drugs in the world. A list of sedative-hypnotics is found in Table 2. Most sedative-hypnotic drugs bind to the GABA receptor complex. The GABA receptor is the most common inhibitory receptor in the central nervous system. There are specific binding sites for the benzodiazepines and the barbiturates on the GABA receptor complex. The benzodiazepines, the most widely prescribed and the safest drugs in this class, are used as anxiolytics (antianxiety drugs), sleeping pills, and muscle relaxants.

TABLE 1

NARCOTIC AGONISTS

MORPHINE
HYDROMORPHONE (DILAUDID)
CODEINE
OXYCODONE (PERCODAN, PERCOCET, ROXYCODONE)
MEPERIDINE (DEMEROL)
METHADONE (DOLOPHINE)
PROPOXYPHENE (DARVON)

MIXED AGONIST-ANTAGONISTS (PARTIAL AGONISTS)

PENTAZOCINE (TALWIN)
NALBUPHINE (NUBAIN)
BUTORPHANOL (STADOL)
BUPRENORPHINE (BUPRENEX)

NARCOTIC ANTAGONISTS

NALOXONE (NARCAN)
NALTREXONE (TREXAN)

TABLE 2

BENZODIAZEPINES

CHLORDIAZEPOXIDE (LIBRIUM)
DIAZEPAM (VALIUM)
OXAZEPAM (SERAX)
TEMAZEPAM (RESTORIL)
CLORAZEPATE (TRANZENE)
TRIAZOLAM (HALCION)
ALPRAZOLAM (XANAX)
PRAZPAM (CENTRAX)

BARBITURATES

SECOBARBITAL (SECONAL)
PENTOBARBITAL (NEMBUTAL)
AMOBARTITAL (AMYTAL)
PHENOBARBITAL (LUMINAL)

SLEEPING PILLS

GLUTETHIMIDE (DORIDEN)
CHLORAL HYDRATE (NOCTEC)
ETHCHLORVYNOL (PLACIDYL)
MEPROBAMATE (EQUANIL)

Both the narcotics and the sedative-hypnotics can cause dependence, and are associated with addictive behavior. Because of this effect, these drugs are under the control of the Controlled Substances Act which places restrictions on how they can be prescribed. There are five classes of drugs in the Controlled Substances act: Class I are drugs that have no legal medical use in the United States (LSD, heroin, mescaline, marijuana, etc.); Class II are drugs that have legitimate medical use but have high abuse potential (cocaine, morphine, amphetamine, and short acting barbiturates); Class III drugs have less abuse potential than Class II, and Class IV drugs have even lower abuse potential. Class V drugs are over the counter drugs that have abuse potential, e.g., certain cough medications. Class I drugs cannot be prescribed. Class II drugs cannot be prescribed for longer than one month, no refills are allowed and prescriptions cannot be conveyed by telephone to the pharmacy. The government can limit the amount of Class II drugs that are manufactured. Class III and IV drug prescriptions can only be written by physicians who have a narcotics license (DEA number).

ASSESSING FOR ADDICTION

Because these drugs have abuse potential, it is important to determine patients who are at risk for addiction and also to monitor carefully patients for whom these drugs are being prescribed to determine if addiction has occurred. One of the best indicators of a potential for addiction is a past history of addiction. This can be ascertained by taking a careful history that includes questions about previous drug use and abuse. The questions should be asked in a matter of fact, nonjudgmental fashion and as part of a regular history from every patient. The questions should include all classes of abused drugs, including dates of use, problems associated with use of drugs, current use and past history of drug abuse treatment. In addition to the patient's history, a family history of drug and alcohol abuse would put the patient at high risk. In taking the family history it is important to go back at least two generations since addiction often skips a generation.

Tolerance is another very important concern with these medications. Tolerance occurs with both narcotics and sedative-hypnotics, and is an adaptation of cells in the body to the presence of the drug resulting in the need to increase the dose in order to achieve the desired effect. Tolerance does not develop to all the effects of the drug at the same rate. Tolerance which develops at different rates to varying effects of the drug is called differential tolerance. An example of this effect is the lack of tolerance to the miotic (pupillary constricting) and constipating effects of narcotics and the rapid onset of tolerance to the sedating and euphoric effects of narcotics. Tolerance develops very slowly to the analgesic effects of narcotics. This differential tolerance can be helpful in determining who is abusing and who is using a narcotic appropriately. In determining how much medication a patient needs to control pain ask the patient, "How much medication do you need to control your pain?" Then give precisely the amount needed to control the pain. If three days later the patient comes back and states that it is not enough medication, then he or she has given an important clue to potential addiction, because tolerance does not develop that rapidly to the analgesic effect of the drug. If, on the other hand, you have underprescribed by giving a low dose of the drug to prevent addiction, then you have no way of knowing who the addict is or who is legitimately seeking the drug for control of pain because you have not given enough to control the pain initially. One of the most common practices with narcotic analgesics is to under-prescribe the drug for fear of respiratory depression. Respiratory depression does not occur as long as the patient is still in pain. If respiratory depression occurs, it is a clue that the pain is under control and the patient may be seeking more drug than needed because of addiction.

Another concern with narcotics and sedative-hypnotics is altered mental status. The benzodiazepines can cause anterograde amnesia. This can be a significant problem during rehabilitation when patients need to recall what they are being taught. Sedative-hypnotics are also effective muscle relaxants and are used to treat contractions. However, this effect and their effect on the cerebellum can result in a loss of coordination that could severely hamper rehabilitation efforts. Thus, there are benefits and liabilities in using these medications. When used sensibly, one can get good results without significant problems.

RULES FOR PRESCRIBING

Unlike some medications where one dose is beneficial to everyone taking the drug, narcotics and sedative-hypnotics have to be titrated carefully to achieve the maximum benefit with the least amount of adverse effects. Because of the problems perceived in using narcotic and sedative-hypnotic medications, the following rules may be helpful.

1. Use an appropriate drug for the problem. Not all pain requires the use of narcotics. Burning or itching pain and phantom limb pain may respond to anticonvulsant medications or antidepressants. It is necessary to take a careful history to characterize the type of pain the patient has in order to prescribe the appropriate medication. Benzodiazepines are now available as short, intermediate and long-acting drugs. Long-acting forms may accumulate in the elderly or in patients with liver impairment. Some benzodiazepines have more specific anxiolytic effects such as alprazolam, and others such as diazepam are better muscle relaxants (DuPont, 1990).

2. Know the pharmacology of the drugs that you are prescribing. How does the drug work and what is its duration of action? If the medication only has a duration of action of three hours, it should not be prescribed every six hours, because the patient will not get a sustained effect. How much drug is necessary to achieve the desired effect? What is the ratio between oral and parenteral doses of the drug?

Many narcotics taken orally are significantly metabolized in the liver before they get to the site of action. This is called first pass metabolism. These drugs require significantly higher doses orally than by injection, sometimes a five- or six-fold difference. Most benzodiazepines, however, are poorly absorbed from intramuscular injection sites and have better absorption when given orally. Some benzodiazepines such as oxazepam, alprazolam, and triazolam are directly metabolized to nonactive compounds, while others such as diazepam and chlordiazepoxide have several active metabolites resulting in a prolongation of their duration of action (Harvey, 1985). Table 3 shows the ratios between oral and parenteral doses of most of the commonly used narcotic medications.

3. Consider prescribing combinations of drugs to increase the effectiveness of the primary drug. If this is done, avoid fixed dose

TABLE 3. Relative Potencies of Analgesics Commonly Employed for Severe Pain Expressed in Terms of the Intramuscular (IM) and Oral (PO) Doses Approximately Equivalent in Total Effect to a 10 mg Dose of Morphine

	IM (mg)	PO (mg)	Major Differences from Morphine
BUPRENORPHINE (Buprinex)	0.3		Partial agonist; longer acting than morphine; in higher doses antagonist effect predominate.
BUTORPHANOL (Stadol)	2		Strong narcotic antagonist action.
CODEINE	130	200	Relatively high PO to IM potency; relatively more toxic in higher doses.
DEXTROPROPOXYPHENE		240	Similar to codeine but more toxic in higher doses.
HEROIN	4		Shorter Acting.
HYDROMORPHONE (Dilaudid)	1.5	7.5	Shorter Acting.

Drug	IM	PO	Comments
LEVORPHANOL (Levodromoran)	2	4	Relatively high PO to IM potency.
MEPERIDINE (Pethidine, Demerol)	75	300	Active metabolite with stimulant properties.
METHADONE (Dolophine)	5	10	Relatively high PO to IM potency, strong sedation, slow onset of analgesia.
METHOTRIMEPRAZINE (Levoprome, Nozinan)	20		Phenothiazine-unlike morphine.
MORPHINE	<u>10</u>	<u>60</u>	
OXYCODONE	15	30	Shorter acting. Relatively high PO to IM potency.
OXYMORPHONE (Numorphan)	1	6	None.
PENTAZOCINE (Talwin)	60	180	Narcotic antagonist analgesic.

combinations because it is frequently necessary to titrate the dose of each drug independently. Often, giving a narcotic and a non-narcotic analgesic drug, such as acetaminophen or aspirin, can be very effective. These two drugs have very different mechanisms of action than the narcotics and can enhance control of pain over the narcotic alone. Combinations of anticonvulsant medications, antidepressants and antipsychotic medications with narcotics can also work very well together. If you are going to give combinations, however, do not give combinations that increase sedation without increasing the effectiveness of the primary drug. There is no fixed dose of narcotic medication that works with everybody. Titrate the dose of the drug to the desired clinical effects to make sure the patient achieves maximum benefit without undue side effects.

4. Narcotic medication should always be given at fixed dosing intervals, not on a PRN schedule. When medication is given on a PRN schedule, the patient must wait until there is pain in order to take the medication. The concept behind the PRN schedule was to reduce the amount of medication the patient takes and reduce the chance of abuse. There are several reasons that this approach doesn't work: (1) addiction is characterized by drug-seeking behavior and PRN schedules reinforce drug-seeking behavior; (2) lower doses of medication are required to maintain the patient in a pain-free state than to stop pain each time it returns; and (3) it is more difficult to determine the patient who is drug-seeking if the medication is given PRN than if the drug is given on a fixed schedule based on the duration of action of the drug. A significant prescribing error is giving the drugs PRN and setting the interval between doses at a time longer than the duration of action of the drug. This mistake strongly reinforces drug-seeking behavior. When patients rightfully try to get medication as the pain returns, a note is placed on the patient's chart, "Patient calling for medication early; must be addicted." Based on the note, someone gets the idea that the best thing to do is inject the patient with saline, because that is going to demonstrate whether or not the patient is truly addicted. So, then you will see a note on the chart that says, "Patient responded to saline, therefore, patient is addicted." Or you will see a note on the chart, "Patient did not respond to saline, therefore, patient is addicted." Consequently, the patient has lost credibility no matter what has happened, and an adversarial relationship is established between the patient and the health care providers. The patient is in pain; the nurses and the physicians are unhappy because they have a difficult patient. All of these events occurred because somebody decided the best way to give this medication is PRN. To summarize, pain medication should be given at a fixed interval, consistent with the duration of action of the medication.

Sedative-hypnotic drugs can be used to treat sleep disorders, spasticity and anxiety disorders. Like any other medication, they should not be used to treat trivial problems, but instead be reserved for patients who have bonafide medical problems. Problems like excessive caffeine intake or short-lived situational problems can be handled with caffeine reduction or counseling. There has been significant concern recently about over-prescribing of benzodiazepines. This is not substantiated by the literature (Woods, Katz, & Winger, 1988; DuPont, 1988). Over the past 15 years the number of benzodiazepine prescriptions has decreased, and there is mounting evidence that, like the narcotics, they may be under prescribed rather than over prescribed. However, since they do have abuse potential, care must be taken in prescribing both narcotics and sedative-hypnotics.

5. Anticipate and treat side effects. Side effects like sedation, constipation, dry mouth, and urinary hesitancy are very common and should be discussed with the patient when the drug is prescribed so they are not surprised. Nausea and vomiting are common when narcotics are first prescribed and tolerance usually develops rapidly to these effects.

6. Monitor for signs of abuse. This is very important, and applies to both classes of drugs. If the patient starts to escalate the dose very rapidly, that is often a sign of abuse. If the patient returns and states that the drug is not effective anymore or suddenly calls to say that he or she has lost the prescription or the dog ate the drugs, or there was a workman in the house who happened to steal the drug from the medicine cabinet, or somebody on the bus took the medication, then these excuses should be regarded as clues that this patient is at high risk for abuse of the drug. Patients who do not have abuse problems never lose their drugs. One way of avoiding problems of excessive medication use is to prescribe just enough medication until the next visit. The patient is informed of this and told to call if there are any problems. This provides information not only on the patient who may be abusing the medication, but also provides information on the patient whose condition is rapidly changing and needs immediate attention. It is also helpful to ask patients to bring any remaining medication to the next visit. This affords information on exactly how much medication the patient is taking. If the patient cannot go one month without abusing the medication, it may be necessary to see the patient weekly or daily until he or she can use the medication in the prescribed manner. As the patient learns to control the use of the medication, then the prescribing interval can be lengthened. Patients with long histories of drug abuse have learned to properly use narcotic and sedative-hypnotic medications without abusing them with this technique.

When there is concern about abuse or addiction, monitoring the patient's urine for the presence of other drugs of abuse and the prescribed drug can be very helpful. There is no need to ask the patient's permission for a urine toxicology outside of the general consent to treatment if the information is part of the confidential doctor-patient relationship. A special consent may be required if the information is to be used for legal or other nonmedical purposes.

Important considerations in prescribing sedative-hypnotics include: (1) titrate the dose of the medication to the needs of the patient; (2) monitor for signs of abuse such as lost prescriptions, rapid escalation of dose, running out of medication early, failure to keep appointments and then calling in for refills; (3) know how to get someone off of the medication if you start to prescribe it; (4) understand the difference between addiction and dependence; and (5) never stop these medications precipitously.

7. *Warn patients about drug interactions.* All of these drugs interact with alcohol. Patients should be told that there are potential problems if they drink or take other medications without letting you know. The most common side effect from these medications is sedation. Use of any other drug that causes sedation can potentiate the sedating effect resulting in severe problems for the patient.

CONCLUSION

Narcotic and sedative-hypnotic drugs are frequently part of the treatment of patients with disabilities of various etiologies. In patients with trauma-induced disabilities, abuse of drugs and alcohol may have played an important part in the traumatic event. Despite the side effects and the potential for abuse by the patient, these drugs should not be denied to patients who need them. A careful history and close monitoring of the patient will alert you to the patient who is at risk or starting to abuse medication. By using the techniques described, these patients can be prescribed the medications they need and their addiction can be controlled. There is no need to deny valuable medication even with addicted patients.

REFERENCES

Cloninger, C.R. (1987). Neurogenetic adoptive mechanisms in alcoholism. *Science, 236,* 410-416.

Cloninger, C.R., Bohman, M. & Sigvardsson, S. (1981). Inheritance of alcohol abuse. *Archives of General Psychiatry, 38,* 861-868.

Diagnostic and Statistical Manual, Third Edition, Revised. (1978). American Psychiatric Association.

DuPont, R.L. (1990). A physician's guide to discontinuing benzodiazepine therapy. *Western Journal of Medicine, 152,* 600-603.

Dupont, R.L. (1988). Abuse of benzodiazepines: The problems and the solutions. *American Journal of Alcohol and Drug Abuse, 14* (Supplement 1).

Goodwin, S.W. & Warnock, J.K. (1991). Alcoholism: A family disease. In Frances & Miller (Eds.) *Clinical Textbook of Addictive Disorders* (pp. 485-500). New York: Guilford Press.

Harvey, S.C. (1985). Hypnotics and sedatives. In Gilman, Goodman, Rall, & Murad (Eds.), *Biological Basis of Therapeutics* (p. 348). New York: Macmillan.

Miller, M.S., Gold, N.S., Belkin, B. & Klahr, A.L. (1989). The diagnosis of alcohol and cannabis dependence in cocaine dependents and alcohol dependence in their families. *British Journal of Addiction, 84,* 1491-1498.

Miller, R.R. & Jick, H. (1978). Clinical effects of meperidine in hospitalized medical patients. *Journal of Clinical Pharmacology, 18,* 180-189.

Porter, J. & Jick, H. (1980). Addiction rare in patients treated with narcotics. *New England Journal of Medicine, 302,* 123.

Woods, J.H., Katz, J. L. & Winger, G. (1988). Use and abuse of benzodiazepines: Issues relevant to prescribing. *Journal of the American Medical Association, 260,* 3476-3480.

Chapter 7

Medical Complications in Rehabilitation

Gary M. Yarkony, MD

Rehabilitation seeks to restore people who have incurred injury or who have a chronic illness to their fullest potential (De Lisa, 1988). This may include physical, psychological, social, vocational, recreational and educational aspects of life. An interdisciplinary team consisting of a physician, nurse, physical therapist, occupational therapist, speech and language pathologist, psychologist, social worker, recreation therapist and vocational rehabilitation counselor is often required for this process. Outcomes may be limited by physical impairments and environmental factors. The purpose of this chapter is to provide an overview of specific traumatic conditions which require rehabilitation, the medical complications, including substance abuse which may impact on these conditions, and the psychosocial consequences of these conditions. The impact of pre-injury adaptation on the rehabilitation process will be discussed.

SPINAL CORD INJURY

There are approximately 10,000 traumatic spinal cord injuries in the United States each year (Anderson & McLaurin, 1980). They are most commonly caused by motor vehicle accidents, sporting injuries such as diving, violence (gunshot and knife wounds) and falls (Stover & Fine, 1986). There is generally an injury to a vertebra resulting in damage to the spinal cord. The damage may improve with time allowing for neural recovery; but generally the more severe the loss of motor and sensory function initially the less the likelihood for recovery. The majority of spinal cord injuries (82%) occur in men, and the average age is approximately 28 years. Many people are under the influence of alcohol or other drugs at the time they sustain these injuries. There are approximately 250,000 individuals in the United States with spinal cord injuries.

Quadriplegia results from injury to the cervical spinal cord. Lesions may be complete or incomplete. Persons with complete lesions have no sensory or motor function below the zone of partial preservation, while persons with incomplete injuries have varying degrees of functional preservation. Cervical injuries result in complete or partial paralysis of the arms and paralysis of the legs. Patients with lesions above the fourth cervical segment may require assistance to breathe. Phrenic nerve pacemakers, an electrical device which stimulates the nerve to the diaphragm, may be used in a limited number of patients with quadriplegia who cannot breathe, but who have the phrenic nerve intact. Other patients with high quadriplegia may require long-term ventilatory support. Rehabilitation of these patients involves training to use electric-powered devices such as wheelchairs, computers and environmental controls by breath or chin controls. Patients with lower level quadriplegia generally use orthotics and other adaptive devices to compensate for muscle weakness. Patients with incomplete syndromes, such as central cord syndrome, may ambulate.

Paraplegia or paraparesis results from injuries to the thoracic, lumber or sacral spinal cord including the conus medullaris and cauda equina (American Spinal Injury Association, 1990). Upper extremity function is preserved and there are varying degrees of leg paralysis. Patients with complete lesions may be independent with a wheelchair. Ambulation with bilateral, long leg braces and crutches is limited due to the marked energy consumption which may be as high as six to 12 times per unit distance that of able-bodied walking.

In addition to the paralysis and loss of sensation accompanying spinal cord injury, neurogenic bowel and bladder dysfunction may result in incontinence. Indwelling catheters, intermittent catheterization, condom (external) catheters and suprapubic catheterization are all options in bladder management. Bowel management may require regular use of stool softeners and suppositories.

Sexual dysfunction is a common sequela of spinal cord injury (Bors & Commarr, 1960; Sha'ked, 1981). This includes both erectile dysfunction and infertility. Women with spinal cord injuries generally resume menstrual function and fertility although pregnancy may be complicated by autonomic dysreflexia.

Diazepam is a drug commonly prescribed to individuals with spinal cord injuries for management of spasticity. It may potentiate depressant effects of alcohol on the central nervous system and must be used with great caution.

TRAUMATIC BRAIN INJURY

There is a wide range of disability which can result from traumatic brain injury (De Lisa, 1988; Yarkony, Betts, & Sahgal, 1983). Most injuries are minor with brief or no loss of consciousness. These injuries may be associated with a post-concussion syndrome. Rehabilitation is generally required in patients with prolonged loss of consciousness. Persons sustaining closed head injury may remain in a persistent vegetative state and never regain meaningful cognitive function although they are not brain dead. They may survive with adequate nursing care. Physical dysfunction may result in hemiplegia or quadriparesis and may be associated with spasticity or ataxia. Cognitive deficits vary from disorders of arousal or attention to loss of higher functions such as memory and integrative function. Behavioral problems such as disruptive or combative behavior may develop. Consequently, some individuals with brain injury may not function appropriately in social situations. The outcomes of these injuries vary widely, with some individuals being paralyzed and dependent on a wheelchair, to individuals who ambulate with minimal cognitive deficits and who behave in a socially appropriate manner.

Drugs acting on the central nervous system are commonly used as post-traumatic epilepsy and behavioral disturbance often occur after brain injury. Great care is necessary in cases of higher functioning persons who drink alcohol because of the risk of drug interactions.

AMPUTATIONS

Amputations of the extremities may result from trauma or disease. Amputations of the upper extremities are generally due to trauma while lower extremity amputations are generally due to disease such as diabetes or peripheral vascular disease. Amputations may occur at the joints (disarticulations), or through the bones of the extremities. Examples of upper extremity amputations are shoulder disarticulations, above elbow, and below elbow amputations. Lower extremity amputations are generally hip disarticulations, above knee and below knee amputations. There are many types of partial foot amputations but the Symes, which is direct end weight bearing, is preferred.

There are two types of control systems for upper extremity prosthesis. Myoelectric devices are electric-powered devices that are activated by a signal from a muscle. These devices are more complex and expensive than standard prostheses that are powered by a device known as a Bowens cable. A harness worn over one or both shoulders supports the prosthesis on the extremity. Movements such as elbow flexion in a below elbow amputation will power a terminal device. Terminal devices may be hooks or cosmetic hands. Hooks are generally more functional, but less cosmetic, and have various designs and sizes for various functions. An example is the farmer's hook.

Lower extremity prostheses have a socket fitted to the extremity and a suspension system. Usually this does not require external straps. There are various knee joints available depending on the stability and activity of the user. Prosthetic feet may vary as well. The Sach foot is used most commonly. Stump socks are used at the interface between the residual limb and the socket. Proper fitting is essential to avoid skin breakdown of the stump.

MEDICAL COMPLICATIONS AFFECTING
REHABILITATION

This section provides an overview of the medical complications which can occur in patients with traumatic injuries during rehabilitation and discusses ways in which substance abuse can exacerbate these complications. These problems are generally secondary to immobilization or to the altered physiology from the neurologic trauma. Although difficult to predict, there is often a tremendous psychological impact. This is particularly true when the complication requires readmission to the acute care hospital where the patient realized the devastation of the initial injury and hoped never to return.

Urinary Tract Infection

During the initial hospital phase, patients being treated for a traumatic injury often have an indwelling catheter placed in their bladder. This allows for drainage of the urinary bladder as well as close monitoring of fluid output. Unfortunately the catheter also is a foreign body in the bladder and serves as a source of infection. Within a short time after catheter insertion, bacteria colonize in the bladder. This may become symptomatic and cause fever. More serious infections may spread to the kidney and are known as pyelonephritis. An infection spreading to the blood, septicemia, will require a prolonged course of antibiotics.

Urinary tract infections may develop in patients who do not empty their bladder completely and regularly (Wu, 1983). Intermittent catheterization decreases the risk of bladder infections although it does not eliminate it completely. Substance abuse may interfere with the ability to follow a catheterization schedule or empty the urinary drainage bag. This may lead to infection or autonomic dysreflexia. In addition, alcohol is a diuretic which, combined with the fluids, may lead to bladder overdistension.

Pneumonia

Pneumonia, a lung infection, is a common complication of immobilization. Immobilized patients often have difficulty clearing secretions from their lungs which may result in infection. Patients with swallowing difficulties may aspirate food into their lungs and develop pneumonia as well. This danger is enhanced by alcohol intoxication. Respiratory therapy and chest physical therapy can be used to expand the lungs and clear secretions. Patients may require tracheostomy to facilitate suctioning. This is often the case in patients with quadriplegia who lose functioning in the chest wall muscles and accessory muscles of respiration. Many of these patients require ventilation temporarily during the acute stage of their injury.

Rehabilitation techniques to improve ventilatory function include incentive spirometry and inspiratory training against progressive resistance (PFLEX). Physical therapy seeks to enhance the strength of the accessory muscles of respiration and maintain mobility of the chest wall. Chest physical therapy mobilizes secretions along with position changes to allow for postural drainage.

Gastrointestinal Complications

Adynamic ileus may develop at the time of acute trauma. This is a frequent complication of abdominal surgery as well. The bowel is temporarily paralyzed and nasogastric suctioning is instituted. As bowel function returns, oral feedings may be reinstituted.

Patients with spinal cord injuries are encouraged to eat a high fiber diet. Stool softeners such as Colace, Senokot or fiber such as Metamucil are often used. Bowel function is generally regulated with suppositories or rectal digital stimulation daily or every other day. This management approach is often used for patients with high paraplegia as well. Patients who sustain distal lesions with flaccid lower motor neuron lesions may require manual removal of feces. Fecal impaction is a common complication. Chronic alcohol abuse may result in constipation which further complicates bowel management. Chronic diarrhea may result from malnutrition.

Bowel infections with organisms such as *Clostridia difficile* may result from repeated use of antibiotics. Duodenal ulceration and bleeding may occur; but it is often prevented by initial nasogastric suctioning and histamine blockers such as Cimetidine or Ranitidine (Matthews & Carlson, 1987; Commarr, 1958).

Pressure Ulcers

Pressure and shear on insensate skin can result in breakdown. These lesions, which in the past were known as decubitus ulcers or bed sores, are now commonly called pressure ulcers or sores. Common sites of these lesions are over the sacral, ischial and greater trochanters. They result from prolonged pressure on skin over bony prominences which causes decreased blood flow and necrosis. Shearing forces, the movement of tissue of different densities upon each other, may decrease the amount of pressure needed to cause ulceration. Skin ulceration is promoted by incontinence and other factors which cause skin macerations. Repetitive mechanical stress may also result in pressure ulcers. Any immobilized person is at risk for pressure ulcer development.

Turning in bed and pressure reliefs while sitting are the mainstay of pressure ulcer prevention. Special air flotation beds may be used both to prevent and treat patients with severe ulceration, but are not a long-term solution. Initially after injury, patients are turned every two hours in bed. This may be increased as skin tolerance develops. If substance abuse inhibits the person's ability to turn, or awareness of the need to turn, the risk of ulceration is increased.

Treatment of pressure ulcers first requires removal of all pressure and debridement of necrotic tissue. This may be done surgically or through use of saline wet-to-dry dressings. Enzymatic preparations for debridement are rarely indicated. Wounds heal faster when placed in a moist environment (Yarkony, Kramer, King, LuKane, & Carle, 1984). Moisture-reactive occlusive dressings, such as Duoderm, are often used. Surgical treatment of deep chronic ulcers, such as those penetrating to bone, is best accomplished through use of a musculocutaneous flap. The bony prominence in the area is removed and adequate soft tissue coverage helps to prevent recurrence. After surgery, sitting is begun when complete wound healing has occurred. Sitting tolerance is increased slowly over several weeks to prevent breakdown of the surgical site.

Kidney and Bladder Complications

Trauma to the nervous system may result in neurogenic bladder dysfunction (Bedbrook, 1979; Borkin, Dolfin, Herschorn, Bhoratwul, & Comisotow, 1983). Patients may initially have a flaccid bladder with urinary retention and require an indwelling Foley catheter. After spinal cord injury, bladder dysfunction may be classified as upper motor neuron (spastic) or lower motor neuron (flaccid). Patients with upper motor neuron bladders may empty reflexively although this is often limited by incoordination between the bladder and sphincter muscles; this condition is known as detrusor sphincter dyssynergia. Patients with flaccid bladders are generally managed by intermittent catheterization. Patients with brain injuries generally regain bladder function. They may, however, have uninhibited bladders caused by a loss of central control which result in frequent voiding of low volumes.

Initial management of trauma patients generally requires an indwelling catheter (Lloyd, Kuhlemeir, Fine, & Stover, 1986). This is often required to monitor fluid output as well as to manage the flaccid bladder. Intermittent catheterization (Guttmann & Frankel, 1966; Kuhlemeir, Lloyd, & Stover, 1985) is generally instituted as soon as feasible. This technique may be continued if bladder function does not return. This technique may be discontinued if reflex voiding occurs with low residual urine. After hospital discharge, patients are generally taught to perform clean catheterization, although sterile intermittent catheterization may be necessary to prevent infection in some individuals. Some patients opt for a suprapubic catheter or indwelling catheter for long-term management, because of convenience or due to an inability to perform catheterization.

Stone formation in the kidneys and bladders is a common complication. Stone formation is more common with indwelling catheterization and infection. Extra-corporeal shock wave lithotripsy has spared many patients the need for surgical intervention to remove kidney stones. Bladder stones are generally removed via a transurethral approach. Dietary modifications limiting calcium intake are suggested to prevent stone formation.

Urethral injuries and penoscrotal fistulas may develop from indwelling catheters. Condom catheters, which are often used in male patients who void without satisfactory control, can lead to skin breakdown and hydronephrosis if applied improperly (Newman & Price, 1985).

Sexual Dysfunction

Loss of erectile function may accompany spinal cord injury (Bors & Commarr, 1960; Sha'ked, 1981). Reflex erections may occur if the sacral cord remains intact. Erectile function is more common with more rostral lesions. Psychogenic erections may be present in patients with distal lesions with the sympathetic outflow intact at the thoracolumbar region. Ejaculation, which may be absent in the presence of erectile function, is more common in patients with incomplete and most distal lesions. Erectile functioning may be restored through vacuum constriction tuminesence therapy or intracorporeal injection of vasoactive substances. Fertility is low, but vibratory or electroejaculation may enhance fertility (Sha'ked, 1981).

Persons sustaining amputations (De Lisa, 1988) due to trauma are primarily limited sexually by phantom pain and problems with psychological adjustment. Body image concerns may limit sexual participation as will problems with the initial adjustment reaction. Advice may be sought in regard to positioning.

Individuals with traumatic brain injury (De Lisa, 1988) may experience sexual dysfunction as part of their social disability. Impulsivity and inappropriate sexual remarks are more common than hypersexuality. Alcohol and other drug abuse may lead to a further disinhibition in these individuals which, in turn, causes further social problems.

Spasticity

Spasticity is a result of injury to the central nervous system (Merritt, 1981) and is a component of upper motor neuron syndrome. Muscle tone is generally diminished following trauma to the central nervous system, but it increases with time. Manifestations of spasticity include increased stretch reflexes and velocity-dependent resistance to passive stretch. Patients with brain injury may initially exhibit decorticate or decerebrate rigidity. Manifestations of spasticity may be part of a picture which includes ataxia from cerebellar lesions. Complications of spasticity include problems with positioning, joint contracture, nursing care and interference with functional activities.

Management of spasticity requires a multifaceted approach. The first step is basic medical care which includes prevention and treatment of pressure sores, bladder stones, and infection. These activities and good passive range of motion exercises may be all that is necessary to prevent spasticity. Spasticity should not necessarily be treated just because it is present; patients should be made aware of this principle. Beneficial effects include decreased lower extremity edema and assistance with standing. Medications include diazepam, Dantrolene, Clonidine, and Baclofen (Davidoff, 1985). Judicious use of diazepam is necessary due to its potential for abuse and interactions with alcohol. Diazepam potentiates the central nervous system depressant of alcohol. Dantrium may cause hepatoxicity. More aggressive management includes nerve blocks, tenotomy or rhizotomy. Baclofen can now be given through an intrathecal pump; this is a major advance in management of severe spasticity. Individuals with a history of drug abuse or alcoholism may be predisposed to developing dependence on diazepam. Prescription of Baclofen and Clonidine should generally be attempted before initiation of diazepam therapy. Prescriptions should be limited to a fixed supply each month to avoid dependence and overmedication.

Heterotopic Ossification

Bone may develop in abnormal locations, most often the hips and knees, after spinal cord or head injury (Stover, Hataway, & Zeiger, 1975; Stover, 1986). Other names for this condition include ectopic bone or paraosteoarthropathy (Kewalramani, 1977). The incidence after spinal cord injury ranges from 16% to 53% and in brain injury from 11% to 76%. Etidronate disodium may be used prophylactically to decrease the amount, but not the incidence, after spinal cord injury.

The dangers of heterotopic ossification include joint contracture deformity which, in turn, can cause pressure sores and interfere with function. Range of motion exercises should be continued after heterotopic ossification develops. Surgical treatment is only indicated for functional interference, pressure sores, or complications of surgery such as bleeding and infection.

Autonomic Dysreflexia

Individuals with spinal cord injuries above the sixth thoracic segment may develop a syndrome of exaggerated sympathetic response to a noxious stimulus below the level of injury (Erickson, 1980). The noxious stimulus is usually bladder or bowel distension but may be tight clothing or leg bag straps, pressure sores or ingrown toenails. The result is hypertension, a pounding headache and symptoms such as piloerection and nasal stuffiness. Morbidity results from the hypertension and can result in seizures, loss of consciousness, intracerebral bleeding and death. Noncompliance with medical regimens may result in an increased risk of dysreflexia.

Intervention begins with sitting the patient upright and removing the cause. Draining a leg bag, unkinking a catheter or straight catheterization usually resolves the problem. If this does not work, antihypertensive medication may be given. Longterm prophylaxis requires alpha blockers such as Prazosin or Dibenzyline.

PSYCHOSOCIAL CONSEQUENCES OF DISABILITY

This paper has briefly reviewed the medical complications that may accompany physical disability and related substance abuse issues. A loss of dignity and privacy, and a reduction in self-image is often associated with traumatic disability. Individuals may assume a "sick role" in their dealings with others. Tremendous coping skills are needed to deal with the primary disability as well as complications such as pressure sores and infection. The individual must learn to deal with health care professionals, decreased independence and must now rely on others for the most basic of needs. They may no longer be able to assume their previous role in a family whose adjustment may be a problem as well. Depression, withdrawal, and isolation are common sequelae. Individuals who are depressed or isolated may develop dependence on drugs and alcohol. This further inhibits reintegration into society and the likelihood of a successful rehabilitation outcome.

The pre-injury adjustment of the individual plays a major role in post-injury outcome. Many patients have a prior history of substance abuse or psychological and medical problems. Often these problems may have contributed to the occurrence of the injury and must be dealt with if rehabilitation is to be successful.

SUMMARY

Drug interactions and substance abuse resulting in secondary disability are a major issue when working with people who have sustained physical disabilities (Gilman, Goodman, Rall, & Murad, 1985). Impaired muscle coordination and judgment resulting from alcohol use is increased in persons who take sedatives, hypnotics, antidepressants, antianxiety drugs, and narcotic analgesics. Acute alcohol intoxication may delay excretion of phenytoin, but chronic usage causes enhanced clearance. Cross tolerance to sedative-hypnotics may develop in alcoholics as well. Tolerance may be pharmacodynamic with a reduced response to the same drug concentration, or dispositional, with decreased duration and intensity of response to a given dose. Tolerance to benzodiazepines results from both pharmacodynamic tolerance and increased rates of metabolism. Individuals tolerant to alcohol may be tolerant to general anesthetics. There is no cross tolerance to alcohol and opiods (Gilman, Goodman, Rall, & Murad, 1985).

Alcohol usage has been noted in our clinical experience to be a cause of secondary disability. This problem may result from alcohol usage alone or in combination with other drugs. Recent studies by Heinemann reveal that 49% of individuals with recent spinal cord injury have heavy drinking histories (Heinemann, Keen, Donohue, & Schnoll, 1988). Falls from wheelchairs have resulted in injuries to the extremities and spine. Gastrointestinal bleeding may occur with diagnosis obscured by the sensory loss. Substance abuse limits reintegration into the community and prohibits use of beneficial medications such as diazepam for spasticity. The individual impaired by drugs or alcohol may develop pressure ulcers while intoxicated. This can result from even one episode of alcohol abuse. A lack of follow-through on required procedures such as intermittent catheterization may lead to infection or autonomic dysreflexia from bladder overdistension. Persons with disabilities are, of course, prone to all other complications of substance abuse experienced by the general population. These complications include degenerative diseases of the nervous system, malnutrition, cardiac disease, liver disease and an increased risk of cancer.

The rehabilitation of individuals with traumatic injuries is a complex task. An interdisciplinary team with expertise from various fields is best suited to this task. Substance abuse as a secondary complication must be recognized quickly and drug interactions identified early in order to minimize morbidity and enhance rehabilitation outcomes. As more and more individuals survive traumatic injuries and live longer lives, the medical and psychosocial consequences of these injuries must be addressed.

REFERENCES

American Spinal Injury Association (1990). *Standards for neurological classification of spinal injury patients.* Chicago: American Spinal Injury Association.

Anderson, D.W., & McLaurin, R.L. (1980). The national head and spinal cord injury survey. *Journal of Neurosurgery, 53,* S1-S43.

Bedbrook, G.M. (1979). Spinal injuries with tetraplegia and paraplegia. *Journal of Bone and Joint Surgery, 61B,* 267-284.

Borkin, M., Dolfin, D., Herschorn, S., Bhoratwul, N., & Comisotow, R. (1983). The urologic care of the spinal cord injury patient. *Journal of Urology, 129,* 335-339.

Bors, E., & Commarr, A.E. (1960). Neurological disturbances of sexual function with special reference to 529 patients with spinal cord injury. *Urological Survey, 10,* 191-222.

Commarr, A.E. (1958). Bowel regulation for patients with spinal cord injury. *Journal of the American Medical Association, 167,* 18-21.

Davidoff, R.A. (1985). Antispasticity drugs: Mechanisms of action. *Annals of Neurology, 17,* 107-116.

De Lisa, J.A. (1988). *Rehabilitation medicine: Principles and practice.* Philadelphia: J.B. Lippincott.

Erickson, R.P. (1980). Autonomic hyperreflexia: Pathophysiology and medical management. *Archives of Physical Medicine and Rehabilitation, 61,* 431-440.

Gilman, A.G., Goodman, L.S., Rall, T.W., & Murad, F. (1985). *The Pharmacological basis of therapeutics* (7th ed.). Macmillan Publishing Company: New York.

Guttmann, L., & Frankel, H. (1966). The value of intermittent catheterization in the early management of traumatic paraplegia and tetraplegia. *Paraplegia, 4,* 63- 83.

Heinemann, A.W., Keen, M., Donohue, R., & Schnoll, S. (1988). Alcohol use by persons with recent spinal cord injury. *Archives of Physical Medicine and Rehabilitation, 69,* 619-629.

Kewalramani, L.S. (1977). Ectopic ossification. *American Journal of Physical Medicine, 56,* 99-120.

Kuhlemeir, K.N., Lloyd, L.K, & Stover, S.L (1985). Long-term follow-up of renal function after spinal cord injury. *Journal of Urology, 134,* 510-513.

Lloyd, L.K., Kuhlemeir, K.V., Fine, P.R., & Stover, S.L. (1986). Initial bladder management in spinal cord injury: Does it make a difference? *Journal of Urology, 135,* 523-527.

Matthews, P.J., & Carlson, C.E. (1987). *Spinal cord injury: A guide to rehabilitation nursing.* Rockville: Aspen.

Merritt, J.L. (1981). Management of spasticity in spinal cord injury. *Mayo Clinic Proceedings, 56,* 614-622.

Newman, E., & Price, M. (1985). External catheters: Hazards and benefits of their use by men with spinal cord lesions. *Archives of Physical Medicine and Rehabilitation, 66,* 310-313.

Sha'ked, A. (1981). *Human sexuality and rehabilitation medicine: Sexual functioning following spinal cord injury.* Baltimore: Williams & Wilkins.

Stover, S.L. (1986). Heterotopic ossification. In R.F. Bloch, & M. Basbaum (Eds.), *Management of spinal cord injuries* (pp. 284-301). Baltimore: Williams and Wilkins.

Stover, S.L., Hataway, C.T., & Zeiger, H.E. (1975). Heterotopic ossification in spinal cord injured patients. *Archive of Physical Medicine and Rehabilitation, 56,* 199-204.

Stover, S.L. & Fine, P.R. (1986). *Spinal cord injury: The facts and figures.* Birmingham: University of Alabama, 1986.

Wu, Y.C. (1983). Total bladder care for the spinal cord injured patient. *Annals of the Academy of Medicine (Singapore), 12,* 387-399.

Yarkony, G.M., Betts, H.B., & Sahgal, V. (1983): Rehabilitation in craniocerebral trauma. *Annals of the Academy of Medicine 12,* 417-427.

Yarkony, G.M., Kramer, E., King, R.B., LuKane, C., & Carle, T.V. (1984). Pressure sore management: Efficacy of a moisture reactive occlusive dressing. *Archives of Physical Medicine and Rehabilitation, 65,* 597-600.

Chapter 8

Pain Management in Rehabilitation

Yvonne Shade-Zeldow, PhD

The scope of the problem of chronic pain in the United States is enormous and continues to expand. Fifteen million Americans suffer chronic pain, with one million new individuals disabled annually by back pain alone (Osterweis, Kleinman, & Mechanic, 1987). The financial costs are staggering, with $50 billion a year and over 400,000 back surgeries annually. Fourteen hundred days of work are lost per 1,000 individual workers due to back injuries alone. Nevertheless, effective treatment of chronic pain problems has often proven to be elusive. Concomitantly, patients have become better informed consumers and have begun to expect to be partners in their health care, often demanding immediate symptomatic relief and cure in the longer term.

Indeed, the largest proportion of individuals who experience pain problems following injury of one sort or another are asymptomatic within months. Unfortunately, by the time rehabilitation centers and programs are typically called upon to evaluate and treat pain patients, their problems have most often become unremitting and chronic. Their histories include numerous interventions, often with multiple surgeries, all of which have failed to completely alleviate their pain. They are, quite literally, at "the end of the road" and facing a peculiar dilemma: still desirous of a cure for their pain problems, they are now encouraged to accept treatment designed to help them live more effectively with pain. Although rehabilitation programs in the United States have slowly moved toward earlier identification and rehabilitation treatment of patients, progress toward this end has often been stymied by financial and institutional disincentives to the infusion of intensive efforts early in the post-injury period.

Fordyce and his colleagues revolutionized the treatment of chronic pain in the late 1960s, when pioneering an operant approach to pain problems (Fordyce, Fowler, & DeLateur, 1968; Fordyce, Fowler, Lehmann, & DeLateur, 1968). These early efforts to programmatically apply behavior modification techniques across all therapeutic disciplines were designed to increase patient activity, to decrease pain-related disability and expressions of pain, and to reduce medication usage for pain control. The application of a behavioral learning model to treatment programs continues to shape programmatic decisions in the vast majority of multidisciplinary pain centers today. Essentially, the primary goal of such programs is to return patients to as normal a lifestyle as possible. To do so, pain is not treated in an attempt to cure, but behavioral methods are used to treat the disabilities and expression of suffering incurred following injury.

While the breadth of goals aspired to by any given pain treatment program may vary (Sternbach, 1974; Fordyce, 1976), multidisciplinary pain programs rather consistently espouse the same basic tenets which are communicated to all patients. All are expected to assume an active role in their own rehabilitation and to collaborate as a partner with therapists, relinquishing the role of passive health care recipient. Second, patients must learn to reconceptualize their pain. One's pain problem is viewed as a life circumstance to be managed rather than a puzzle for someone to diagnose and cure. This hallmark of pain centers is neatly woven through all aspects of clinically respected programs, yet it is a tenet not eagerly embraced by every patient. The struggle to accept less than complete comfort and physical functioning is played out daily in the course of any treatment program. The issue of learning to control pain and limit its negative impact on daily living becomes the focus of even the most mundane moments of treatment.

Additionally, therapists across all disciplines focus with the patient on developing effective means of coping with pain and altered life circumstances. This most often translates as well into confronting and replacing negative, maladaptive behavior patterns and pain behaviors which have been utilized by the patient in the communication of his discomfort. While the techniques employed within the context of each program and treatment modality may vary (Cairns, Thomas, Mooney, & Pace, 1976; Kerns, Turk, & Holzman, 1983), the theoretical underpinnings consistently assume that chronic pain has developed at least in part because pain behaviors (verbal and nonverbal) that began in response to an acute injury have been met with positive consequences. Therefore, identifying and removing reinforcers that have served to contribute to dysfunction and to maintain pain behavior, while simultaneously promoting and reinforcing well behaviors is the keystone to pain management.

A number of techniques are traditionally used in most pain treatment programs, with modifications as elected or required by a particular setting. They include exercise programs done to quota rather than tolerance, inattention to pain behaviors, interpersonal support and attention to well behaviors, restorative vocational efforts, pacing of physical activity, and family training and involvement to support consistent and appropriate follow through in the return to the home environment. Lastly, medication withdrawal is routinely addressed and managed in most pain management programs through use of operant principles.

Specific operant techniques employed in pain programs are many. For success to occur, however, consistent application of whatever techniques are chosen to meet patient goals is critical.While creative means to reach goals, such as greater function despite pain, return to work, and the like are to be lauded, it is not the number of techniques applied that produces results. The careful and consistent integration of behavioral principles and techniques across all modalities (i.e., physical therapy, occupational therapy, nursing) will maximize success. Indeed, it is on this plane that programs face their most difficult challenge. Fordyce was well aware, from his first observations, of how pervasive and entrenched patient (and family) behaviors in response to pain could be, requiring an intensive effort to induce change on any functional dimension.

Medication use itself in chronic pain patients is fraught with a number of potential iatrogenic factors. These particular patients are frequently prescribed narcotic analgesics with high abuse potential.

Second, it is extremely common to prescribe these analgesics on an as needed (PRN) basis. Many patients report becoming preoccupied with their physical state in order to justify taking more medication. Anxiety and fear may lead to medication use in anticipation that the pain will get much worse or simply to avoid this possibility. These same patients also quickly acknowledge that, with chronic usage, medication rarely does more than take the edge off. Despite this self-assessment, they are fearful to be left without medication within easy reach.

While prescription drug usage is addressed at length in Dr. Schnoll's chapter, several comments in the context of chronic pain are in order. Although the motivation to prescribe analgesics, muscle relaxants, etc., on a PRN basis is primarily to limit use to times when the medication is essential, the reality is that writing and renewing prescriptions is a relatively expedient means to temporarily satisfy an already frustrated and needy pain patient. It also reduces the likelihood of additional office visits and phone calls asking for help in the immediate future. Lack of appropriate and consistent follow-up communication between physician and patient around medication usage is not unusual. Therefore, we often see appropriate medication being used inappropriately and without guidance or supervision.

Helping patients gain control over a medication regimen that has gone awry occurs when, within the context of a rehabilitation program, medication use is made contingent not upon increased pain but upon time. Pain cocktails (Fordyce, 1976), or some variant of this approach, are often used with full knowledge and consent of patients. Many programs require this component in treatment of all analgesic using patients. Toward the goal of weaning patients from medication, the amount of active agent (medicine) is tapered over time, usually within a controlled amount of flavored elixir or juice. Patients understand time-contingent usage quite quickly. They also are able to observe here the discrepancy between their anticipated, fearful response and actual outcome, which is most often that they, indeed, do not feel worse. Most important, this approach encourages and reinforces a sense of patient control rather than reliance on external means to alter discomfort.

In rehabilitation, one additional feature of medication use and reduction is important to note. It is all too frequently the case that, within several weeks of discharge, patients return for checkup appointments reporting return to prior medication use, even to PRN usage. These circumstances follow intensive instruction, prior patient cooperation and good clinical results. Needless to say, this state of affairs is discouraging and frustrating for professional staff. It does, however, point to an issue which we need to attend to more consistently. Following specialty programmatic treatment, patients are routinely referred back, or return on their own, to their primary physicians. The recidivism we observe reflects in large part a confluence of newly achieved yet fragile gains in the patient and a physician who has not usually participated in any aspect of the patient's course of treatment. Thus, while the physician may be quite pleased with what he sees, he is as likely as before to prescribe in the fashion of previous experience. Hence, unless we commit ourselves to consistently educating within the realm of the local community and private practice, we will continue to have our therapeutic efforts thwarted, albeit unintentionally.

As Turk and Flor (1987) note, failure to consider psychosocial factors may result in both an inadequate understanding of pain patients and unnecessarily limited results. Given an operant paradigm within which to function professionally, it can be all too easy to grow inattentive to how anxiety, depression and preoccupation with pain have heightened the impact of pain on overall adjustment. Spousal reactions, marital satisfaction and satisfaction with social support clearly relate to pain behavior (Block, 1980; Gil, Keefe, Crisson, & Van Dalfsen, 1987). Counseling aimed toward enhancing the patient's ability to cope has a positive effect on overall functioning. Teaching patients to discriminate between those coping responses effective in the short term from those most likely to be effective in the long term will enhance both sense of control and level of function.

While the operant schema emphasizes the role of environmental factors in maintaining pain behavior and limited function, the cognitive-behavioral approach focuses on the ways in which beliefs, thoughts and expectations contribute to patients' behavior and emotional response to pain (Turner & Chapman, 1982; Pearce, 1983). Here, the therapeutic focus is on the patient's means of interpreting and thinking about painful experience, which is often maladaptive and adds to the negative impact of pain. Such cognitive distortions and erroneous attributions are thought to cause patients to experience depression, anxiety and hopelessness, therein resulting in excessive suffering. Through group and individual therapy, a cognitive-behavioral focus assists patients in reinterpreting their own roles and control over their situations, to put into place a more accurate framework from which to operate and appraise.

The trend toward outpatient multidisciplinary pain programs, rather than hospital- or inpatient-based, has grown in recent years. While the primary motivation for such a shift is improved cost effectiveness, there are also a number of significant treatment benefits. While an outpatient program places clear limits on staff ability to control behavioral contingencies, it also presents for the patient a treatment base which does not artificially remove the realities and stresses of his or her daily life. A by-product of this arrangement is the healthy struggle for each patient to receive help in the context of the real world, not a milieu created especially for him or her. The tension produced by this conflict results, when successful, in a more confident individual who is assured that pain can be managed more capably and its interference in life can be reduced. Additionally, the often seen anxiety heightened at the time of discharge is dramatically reduced when the sudden shift from hospital to home environment is avoided. Encouraging realistic expectations of self and others is inherently useful in the context of pain management, and experience with this focus within a naturalistic environment is preferable.

Multidisciplinary pain programs seek a synergistic treatment effect. No matter which theoretical base is elected, the integration of sound psychological principles across all disciplines and treatment modalities should maximize therapeutic outcome. Individualized treatment planning attempts to finely hone the skills needed by each patient to achieve greater function and a more limited impact of chronic pain on daily life. By teaching patients that they themselves can be significant agents in controlling pain and its consequences, we have empowered a significantly large population who can again become productive citizens and contribute as active, capable adults. Our goal for the future, nonetheless, must be consistent attention to these issues and potential treatment more actively following injury, such that remedication is relatively swift and effective, both in terms of financial and personal cost to all involved in the chronic pain arena.

REFERENCES

Block, A.R. (1980). An investigation of the response of the spouse to chronic pain behavior. *Psychosomatic Medicine, 43*, 415-422.

Cairns, D., Thomas, L., Mooney, V., & Pace, J.B. (1976). A comprehensive treatment approach to chronic low back pain. *Pain, 2*, 302-308.

Fordyce, W.E. (1976). *Behavioral methods in chronic pain and illness*. St. Louis: C.V. Mosby.

Fordyce, W.E., Fowler, R.S., Lehmann, J., & DeLateur, B. (1968). Some implications of learning in problems of chronic pain. *Journal of Chronic Disease, 21*, 179-190.

Fordyce, W.E., Fowler, R., & DeLateur, B. (1968). An application of behavior modification technique to a problem of chronic pain. *Behaviour Research and Therapy, 6*, 105-107.

Gil, K.M., Keefe, F.J., Crisson, J.E., & Van Dalfsen, P.J. (1987). Social support and pain behavior. *Pain, 29*, 209-217.

Kerns, R.D., Turk, D.C., & Holzman, A.D. (1983). Psychological treatment for chronic pain: A selective review. *Clinical Psychology Review, 3*, 15-26.

Osterweis, M., Kleinman, A., & Mechanic, D. (1987). *Pain and Disability: Clinical, Behavioral, and Public Policy Perspectives*. Washington, DC: Institute of Medicine, National Academy Press.

Pearce, S. (1983). A review of cognitive-behavioral methods for the treatment of chronic pain. *Journal of Psychosomatic Research, 27*, 431-440.

Sternbach, R.A. (1974). *Pain patients: Traits and treatment*. New York: Academic Press.

Turk, D.C., & Flor, H. (1987). Pain > pain behaviors: The utility and limitations of the pain behavioral construct. *Pain, 31*, 277-295.

Turner, J.A., & Chapman, C.R. (1982). Psychological interventions for chronic pain: A critical review. II. Operant conditioning, hypnosis, and cognitive-behavioral therapy. *Pain, 12*, 23-46.

PART III:
ASSESSMENT, TREATMENT, AND PREVENTION ISSUES

Chapter 9

Substance Abuse Assessment and Treatment: Where We Are, Where We Are Going, and How It Will Affect Services to Persons with Substance Abuse Problems

Thomas J. Budziack, PhD

The substance abuse treatment field is entering a period of uneasy transition. In just the last five years, behavioral science research has raised fundamental questions about how addictions should be conceptualized and treated, challenging some of the longstanding assumptions regarded as fact by many clinicians. These challenges reflect far more than the intellectual meandering of academic theorists; they have clear and important implications for the most fundamental clinical question: Are persons with substance abuse problems receiving the type of treatment most likely to help them manage their problems? Rehabilitation professionals who understand these issues will be able to help clients with substance abuse problems gain access to the most appropriate intervention for each individual's needs.

SUBSTANCE ABUSE TREATMENT TODAY: WHERE WE ARE

Substance abuse treatment today is best characterized by model exclusivity: the predominance of one treatment model that is deemed the "one best way" to treat addictions. The traditional model follows a disease conceptualization paired with Twelve-Step principles of recovery. The disease concept, purportedly based on the pioneering research of Jellinek (1946) and contemporary biomedical researchers, maintains that it is scientifically valid and therapeutically advantageous to define and treat substance abuse as a disease. The Twelve-Step model of recovery, which evolved from the personal experiences of Alcoholics Anonymous members, asserts that persons addicted to alcohol or other drugs must follow a prescribed sequence of activities and experience a spiritual reawakening in order to initiate recovery.

The traditional approach is followed almost universally by American substance abuse treatment programs. Most are firmly committed to the traditional approach as not only the best way but the *only* way to treat addictions. This one best way assumption is so firmly entrenched that some treatment programs exclude any treatment procedures that are not derived from the traditional approach. Consequently, for the vast majority of persons referred to treatment, the traditional disease/Twelve-Step treatment is the only option available.

This chapter will critically evaluate some of the assumptions and beliefs underlying the traditional approach, focusing on those which have direct and important clinical implications. The purpose is *not* to denounce or attack the traditional approach, but rather to evaluate the belief that it is the best and only way to treat addictions. There is no question that millions of people have benefited from traditional treatment; there is little doubt that for some people the Twelve-Step model is the best and perhaps only path to recovery. This chapter addresses another question: Can we be so confident of the universal applicability and effectiveness of the traditional approach that we should follow it to the exclusion of all other approaches? In clinical terms, should substance abuse treatment programs *restrict* treatment options, insisting that all clients follow the traditional approach, or should they *expand* treatment options by offering individualized treatment incorporating a variety of empirically-tested treatment alternatives?

While traditional practitioners frequently cite research to support the one best way assumption and model exclusivity, most of the traditional treatment procedures derive from a craft orientation rather than a scientific model based on systematic investigation. The craft orientation implies that substance abuse counseling skills are best acquired through experiential learning, preferably through experiencing addiction and initiating recovery through a Twelve-Step program. Clinical wisdom gleaned from this experience is usually valued more highly than familiarity with research literature evaluating the effectiveness of treatment procedures.

It is not surprising, then, that recovering counselors play a key role in traditional treatment. Many traditional treatment programs prefer to use recovering counselors, many of whom have limited formal training but rely instead on their own experience as a recovering addict to guide their therapeutic activities.

Many craft-oriented practitioners express a frank disdain for theories and research. There is a vast scientist-practitioner gap in substance abuse treatment, with roots tracing back to the 1930s. In those days, relatively few health professionals were willing to work with substance abusers. Those who did typically interpreted addictive behavior in psychodynamic terms, treating drinking as the symptom of an underlying psychopathology traceable to early childhood experiences. Alcoholics quite correctly saw little relationship between the psychodynamic talk therapies and their here-and-now drinking problem, and turned to mutual self-help groups as a source of more practical, pragmatic help. The Twelve-Step movement was to a large extent a response to ineffectual helping professionals, resulting in a distrust of behavioral science and "psychologizing" that persists today.

Despite claims of proven approaches, most traditional treatment procedures are based on clinicians' personal experiences and preferences rather than objective evidence from controlled research. Dr. Enoch Gordis, director of the National Institute of Alcohol Abuse and Alcoholism, has termed alcoholism treatment "a haphazard mixture of largely unvalidated approaches," noting that ". . . our whole treatment system . . . is founded on hunch, not evidence, and not on science" (1987, p. 582). The next section discusses the important clinical implications of this situation.

BELIEFS, ASSUMPTIONS, CLINICAL IMPLICATIONS

As with any intervention approach, there is a set of beliefs and assumptions underlying the traditional approach. These beliefs and assumptions have a strong influence on the types of procedures used in treatment and how those procedures are applied.

Several traditional beliefs can be subsumed under *the homogeneity assumption:* the notion that people who are alcoholics and/or addicts share common characteristics. The first is the belief that there is a disease, a unitary phenomenon, called alcoholism or addiction. It is believed that people either have the disease–and are alcoholics and/or addicts–or they do not. Alcoholics and addicts are believed to be essentially different from nonaddicts, with "an unidentified, otherwise unspecified lesion somewhere in the body that is responsible for crucial differences in how prealcoholics and others respond to alcohol" (Nathan, 1986, p. 10). Inheritance studies are cited as evidence that this difference is inborn and genetic.

The traditional approach also assumes that the disease has a known course and progression. The so-called "Jellinek curves" which appear throughout the substance abuse literature are widely cited as scientific verification for this assumption. These curves are believed to represent the inexorable progression of the disease, showing that the addict will pass predictable landmarks such as blackouts and loss of control. This curve is cited as evidence that all addicts will eventually hit bottom and either begin recovery or eventually die from the disease.

The traditional approach also assumes that alcoholics and other addicts have predictable traits and common "character defects." Johnson (1980), in a classic text still regarded as authoritative by many substance abuse counselor training programs, declares

> Very different sorts of people become alcoholic, but all alcoholics are ultimately alike. The disease swallows up all differences and creates a *universal alcoholic profile.* The personality changes that go with the illness are predictable and inevitable, with some individual adaptation . . . [but] the classic description fits almost any individual alcoholic to a startling degree. (p. 5, emphasis in the original)

Johnson cites no research to support this far-reaching opinion, apparently basing it on his personal observations. In a similar vein, Hazelden, a treatment center with a prominent role in the development of the traditional model, publishes a series of pamphlets with titles such as *Pride, Perfectionism, Grandiosity, Stinking Thinking,* and *King Baby* describing traits believed to characterize alcoholics. The trait considered most pervasive is denial, described as a pathological addiction-induced inability to be honest with oneself and acknowledge addiction and its concomitant problems.

The homogeneity assumption exerts a major influence on clinical practice. Since it is believed that alcoholism or other addiction is a unitary disease–you have it or you do not–assessment procedures are directed towards a binary diagnosis: alcoholic/addicted or not. For example, the Michigan Alcoholism Screening Test (Selzer, 1971) is typically interpreted using a cutoff score to distinguish alcoholics from nonalcoholics.

Once it is determined that a person is an alcoholic or addict, treatment is diagnosis driven. As Blume (1983) states, characteristics of the individual are not nearly as important as the diagnosis:

> [The traditional approach] searches for common signs and symptoms of disease in individuals (*rather than focusing on the uniqueness of each person*) and uses these common features to establish a diagnosis. The diagnosis, then, allows one to predict a probable course and prognosis . . . . It is only after establishing the diagnosis that the specific gender, ethnic characteristics and circumstances of the individual become important in formulating the treatment plan. (pp. 15-16; parenthetical is from the source, emphasis added)

Since alcoholics/addicts are believed to share common traits and to have common needs, there is a *core treatment* which is presumed necessary for all. As Filstead (1984) notes, this approach predetermines clients' needs on the basis of their diagnosis rather than developing an intervention to fit the individual:

> Patients receive the services the treatment programs offer. . . . Most professionals . . . have assumed their patients form a

homogeneous group and consequently make little effort to differentially assess each patient's needs and recommend treatment based on this assessment. . . .

Organizations assume that their services and programs are appropriate for the patients they treat. . . .

. . . the suggestion to 'determine services based on patient need' may make little sense. This is precisely the problem. If a program has already determined what its patients' needs are, it need not explore this question. (pp. 49-50)

According to this orientation, everyone diagnosed as an alcoholic or addict requires a similar treatment protocol. This is clearly reflected in the program schedules followed by traditional treatment programs. All clients are expected to follow a standard core regimen of predominantly group activities–lectures, group discussion, group therapy, films and videotapes, and Twelve-Step meetings–based on the assumption that all clients have similar needs. While some treatment programs profess to offer individualized treatment, the great majority of treatment hours are devoted to a standard set of pre-programmed group activities.

Another set of critical assumptions and beliefs revolve around *motivation* for treatment. Traditional treatment programs typically assume that resistance to change is based on denial, which in turn is a symptom of addictive disease. Unless denial is aggressively confronted, it is assumed that the addict will be incapable of making informed decisions and will continue to resist treatment. Techniques such as the confrontational intervention, in which the addict is confronted by family and friends in a caring but assertive way, are believed to break through denial and instill motivation to enter treatment.

Officially, Twelve-Step groups are considered a fellowship with a set of guiding principles rather than a form of treatment. However, Twelve-Step principles play an integral if not dominant role in most treatment programs, and it is often difficult to distinguish treatment activities from Twelve-Step activities. In fact, some treatment programs acknowledge that their primary purpose is to introduce patients to Twelve-Step principles and initiate their participation in meetings which are part of the treatment regimen. Consequently, the assumptions and beliefs inherent in the Twelve-Step orientation exert a strong influence on the type of clinical procedures and approaches incorporated into substance abuse treatment.

The Twelve-Steps of Alcoholics Anonymous are listed in Table 1 of Chapter 10. Six of the steps refer to a higher power or God. The reference to God "*as we understood him*" is intended to acknowledge that for some people God or the higher power may be fellowship or some other spiritual value rather than a deity as conceptualized by organized religions. Regardless of the precise nature of the higher power, spirituality plays a prominent role in Twelve-Step processes and persons following a Twelve-Step program must be amenable to that orientation.

The Twelve Steps also require participants to adopt an attitude of submissiveness and humbleness. Several steps demand recognition of powerlessness, turning over will and life to a higher power, asking the higher power to remove shortcomings, and seeking through prayer and meditation to understand "His will for us" (Alcoholics Anonymous World Services, 1976). To successfully follow the Steps, individuals must be open to self-disclosure, willing to confess their wrongs to others, and willing and able to affiliate with the group, which is deemed a potent force in recovery. Since participation in Twelve-Step meetings requires that members explicitly acknowledge their addiction, treatment programs often invest heavily in activities designed to break through denial and force the patient to accept the alcoholic or addict self-label.

The widespread use of recovering counselors also has important clinical implications. While there is no doubt that recovering people have a unique insight into the recovery process and that they could serve as powerful role models for their clients, there are potential problems as well. First, some recovering individuals feel that their personal experience is an adequate and sufficient education for clinical practice; consistent with the craft orientation, many do not see a need to obtain graduate training in a professional discipline. Instead, many seek alcoholism or substance abuse counselor certification which is administered by state boards. However, the educational prerequisites for counselor certification are surprisingly minimal. For example, the Illinois Certification Board's educational requirement for certification is only 100 clock hours, 60 in counseling, 40 in alcoholism. This can be satisfied through junior college certificate programs which do not require an associate's degree as prerequisite.

While the attainment of a professional degree does not ensure clinical competence, the minimal educational requirements for substance abuse counselor certification raises serious questions about their basic skill levels. Once certified, substance abuse counselors may perform assessments, individual and group counseling, and family therapy without having completed any graduate level courses in these areas. The basic skills training provided to substance abuse counselors certainly does not compare to that received by professionals who have earned their master's or doctoral degree.

More important, recovering counselors who fervently adhere to the one best way ideology can impede treatment individualization. The belief that it worked for me, coupled with a personal devotion to the Twelve Steps, often compels counselors to insist that their clients follow the same path. Rather than viewing clients as individuals who might have needs quite different from their own, some recovering counselors see each client as mirroring their own past. The counselor's prescriptions all too often reflect what worked for the counselor instead of what is most likely to work for the client. If recovering counselors resist or reject clinical procedures or approaches which are inconsistent with their own recovery experience, the treatment program's clinical repertoire is narrowed, and clients who could benefit from other paths to sobriety are not offered alternatives.

The clinical implications which follow from a program's treatment philosophy are very real. The beliefs and assumptions underlying a model dictate the kinds of clinical activities that are or are not incorporated into treatment. The obvious next question is "Are a program's assumptions and beliefs supported by objective research evidence?"

RESEARCH EVIDENCE: ARE THE FACTS REALLY PROVEN?

Those who are committed to the traditional approach as the one best way frequently refer to proven facts that validate their views about how substance abuse is best treated. However, many of those views are not supported by evidence from controlled scientific research. Two questions are particularly important from the clinician's perspective: (1) Does research support the homogeneity assumption and the corollary belief that all alcoholics/addicts require the same core treatment, and (2) Is it in fact proven that traditional treatment is the most effective approach?

The Homogeneity Assumption

Biomedical and genetics research is often cited to support the belief that alcoholics and addicts are fundamentally different from non-addicts. For example, it is widely believed that alcoholism is an inherited disease and that medical research will eventually find the long sought-after marker–the hypothesized biological quirk that makes alcoholics or other addicts different from other people.

Is Alcoholism Hereditary?

Mueller and Ketcham (1987) offer an example of the conventional wisdom:

> Alcoholism is passed from alcoholic parents through a genetic susceptibility to alcohol. How do we know this? The best evidence comes from a series of studies conducted by researcher Donald Goodwin. (p. 12, emphasis added)

Goodwin and his associates conducted landmark studies (Goodwin, Schulsinger, Hermansen, Guze, & Winokur, 1973; Goodwin, Schulsinger, Moller, Hermansen, Winokur, & Guze, 1974) in which sons of alcoholics were compared to sons of nonalcoholics where both groups had been adopted in infancy. They found that the children of alcoholics were more likely to develop alcohol problems even when reared apart from their alcoholic parent. This research has commonly been interpreted to suggest that an individual's genetic makeup is more important than environmental influences in determining whether someone will develop a drinking problem.

Mueller and Ketcham's unequivocal proclamation that we *know* alcoholism is inherited stands in marked contrast to Goodwin's interpretation of his own research. Goodwin's (1988) recent book is cautiously worded; he presents his findings conservatively and with careful qualification. For example, in a section highlighted in italics Goodwin states that his research "suggests that severe forms of alcohol abuse may have a genetic predisposition but that heavy drinking itself . . . reflects predominantly nongenetic factors" (p. 107). Goodwin goes on to state that "It should be emphasized that 'genetic predisposition' remains more probable than proven, and certainly may not apply to all alcoholics" (p. 107).

To say that it is probable but not proven that certain severe forms of alcohol abuse may be genetically predisposed is a far cry from knowing that alcoholism is passed from alcoholic parents through a genetic susceptibility to alcohol. Furthermore, Goodwin's analysis of drinking problems among female adoptees produced results markedly different from the findings among male subjects, leading Goodwin to conclude that "From this study, it appears that alcoholism in women may have a partial genetic basis, but the sample size precluded any definitive conclusion" (1988, p. 111).

Goodwin (1988) further qualifies his findings by differentiating between familial and nonfamilial types of alcoholism. He explicitly states that his conclusions about heritability do not apply to the nonfamilial alcoholics (pp. 32-33). He further states that "not everything that runs in families is hereditary" (p. 7) and that it is by no means proven that alcoholism is an inherited disease. Referring to the title of his 1988 book, Goodwin notes "That's why the question mark remains after *Is alcoholism hereditary?*" (p. 156).

Today, few would argue against the likelihood of a genetic component to alcoholism, i.e., that a genetic predisposition contributes to the development of alcoholism in some cases. More recent genetics research, however, is identifying subtypes of alcoholics and does not support the notion of alcoholism as a monolithic unitary disease (Blum et al., 1990; Zucker, 1986). Research by Cloninger and his associates (Bohman, Cloninger, von Knorring, & Sigvardsson, 1984; Cloninger, 1983), for example, suggests that there may be different types of alcoholism which may reflect major differences in genetic contribution. Cloninger's group identified one group manifesting what they termed Type I alcoholism, which was by far the more prevalent type. It was found in both men and women and was marked by onset during adulthood and less severe problems. Type II alcoholism was found only in men and accounted for only 25% of male alcoholics in Cloninger's studies. It was marked by an early onset and more severe social problems related to alcohol use. Cloninger's work suggests that Type II alcoholism is highly influenced by genetics and relatively unaffected by environment; alcohol abuse was nine times more likely among Type II alcoholics regardless of their postnatal environment. Type I alcoholism, on the other hand, seems more environmentally determined, with genetic factors apparently of minor importance (von Knorring, von Knorring, Smigan, Lindberg, & Edholm, 1987).

The "fact" that alcoholism is inherited has been used to support the homogeneity assumption, implying that alcoholics are a distinct subpopulation with a genetically determined flaw that differentiates them from nonalcoholics. Genetics research has been cited as scientific proof of the existence of a unitary disease, and treatment programs have assumed that alcoholics share a genetic flaw which, in turn, dictates the need for a universal core treatment.

In fact, however, heritability and genetic susceptibility remains a hypothesis to be studied, hardly a proven fact (Schuckit, 1987). If anything, the results of genetics research argue against the homogeneity assumption. The dogma that alcoholics are a homogeneous group who have the same disease is being replaced by mounting evidence that there are multiple subtypes with decidedly different characteristics and needs (Zucker, 1986).

The Course and Progression of Addiction

Jellinek's (1946, 1952, 1960) pioneering research is cited as evidence that alcoholics follow a known and predictable path or progression. Glatt (1958) depicted Jellinek's findings in a U-shaped curve which has become ubiquitous in the substance abuse field, appearing in texts, counselor training programs, and as a clinical aid used to explain progression to clients. At least one treatment program has adapted the same U-shaped curve to describe the progression of cocaine addiction and family co-dependency even though there is no evidence this author could locate which suggests that cocaine abusers or family members follow this curve.

In fact, it is difficult to find credible evidence that alcoholics follow the progression depicted in the so-called Jellinek curve. Jellinek (1960) himself repeatedly described his work as a working hypothesis, a theory designed to spur further research, a plausible explanation in need of scientific testing. Pattison, Sobell, and Sobell (1977) believe that Jellinek never intended that his theory be interpreted as a factual description of how alcoholics behave; they describe his 1960 treatise as "a series of working hypotheses clothed in a suit of caveats" (p. 13). Jellinek repeatedly cautioned his readers to distinguish attractive theories from proven fact: "Acceptance of certain formulations on the nature of alcoholism does not necessarily equal validity," he noted, reminding readers that "for the time being, this [his research] may suffice, but not indefinitely" (Jellinek, 1960, p. 159).

Pattison, Sobell, and Sobell (1977) and Fingarette (1988) provide more detailed reviews of the shortcomings of the research behind the curve. To summarize their critiques, the major problem was a small, unrepresentative sample: Ninety-eight male Alcoholics Anonymous members. According to Fingarette, "Jellinek . . . excluded all questionnaires filled out by women because their answers differed greatly from the men's" (p. 21). Jellinek himself explicitly stated that his sample size was small and not representative: "The subject of this study represents not more than a small section of the problems of alcohol–a very small section indeed" (1960, p. ix).

Since 1960, many more rigorous studies have investigated the natural history of alcohol abuse and alcoholism (e.g., Cahalan & Room, 1974; Clark & Cahalan, 1976; Fillmore, 1975; Fillmore & Midanik, 1984; Polich, Armor, & Braiker, 1981; Vaillant, 1983; Wilsnack, Wilsnack, & Klassen, 1986). Not one of these studies confirms the validity of the U-shaped curve; in fact, most flatly contradict Jellinek's progression hypothesis. In particular, the notion of an inexorable downward progression and hitting bottom is not supported; instead, many drinkers with severe problems, including diagnosed alcoholics, can mature out of their drinking patterns without seeking treatment or joining a Twelve-Step group (Cahalan & Room, 1974; Fillmore, 1975; Institute of Medicine, 1990; Mulford, 1984; Vaillant, 1983).

Contrary to the homogeneity assumption, modern research provides a compelling argument against the assumption that alcoholics follow a predictable path or progression. Despite Jellinek's caveats about his own research and decades of disconfirming research, many treatment programs still treat the U-shaped curve as proven fact. On the basis of data nearly a half century old, from a very limited and biased sample, many substance abusers today are being told with certainty that they will follow the same course, despite controlled, contemporary research indicating that this is not necessarily true.

Is There a "Universal Alcoholic Profile?"

The idea that alcoholics share common personality traits and character defects has been cited to support the homogeneity assumption. As Blane and Leonard (1987) point out, however, this is "a point of view" rather than a "coherent body of theory" (p. 5). While the notion of a "universal alcoholic profile" is well-established within clinical folklore (Johnson, 1980) that is not the case among researchers: "Few writers have claimed that all addicts are endowed with a common tragic flaw or the same constellation of weaknesses" (Sutker & Allain, 1988, pp. 174-175).

There is no evidence of a single personality type among persons who abuse alcohol and other drugs (Graham & Strenger, 1988; Nathan, 1988) and the search for "the alcoholic personality" has been abandoned by most behavioral scientists (Cox, 1987). Contemporary research is leaning towards complex multilevel causal chains rather than simplistic "global" explanations of addictive behavior (Blane & Leonard, 1987).

Modern research suggests that people who abuse alcohol and other drugs differ along clinically important dimensions. Skinner (1982) employed the *Alcohol Use Inventory* to identify meaningful differences in drinking *styles*, perceived *benefits* of drinking, type and severity of *consequences* of drinking, *concerns* about the effects of drinking, and *acknowledgment* of a problem. Horn, Wanberg, and Foster (1987) show how these differences can be used to tailor an individualized treatment plan that addresses specific client needs.

Prochaska and his associates (Prochaska & DiClemente, 1986)

have proposed an empirically derived model of the change process that suggests another dimension of differences among alcoholics and addicts. Prochaska's research suggests that an individual may be in any of four stages of readiness to change. In the *Precontemplation* stage, the individual does not perceive his or her substance use as a problem that needs to be addressed. Persons in the *Contemplation* stage perceive the problem but are not convinced that they need to take any action. In the *Action* stage, people are ready to actively problem-solve. During the *Maintenance* stage, people are mainly concerned with preventing relapse. Prochaska's research suggests that interventions should be matched to each individual's stage of change, because people in different stages require fundamentally different interventions. Interventions that are effective with those in the action stage, for example, are not likely to be effective with precontemplators, and vice versa.

Annis' research (Annis & Davis, 1989) demonstrates another way that people who abuse alcohol and other drugs can differ. Annis and her associates were inspired by Marlatt's research on relapse prevention (Marlatt & Gordon, 1985). According to Marlatt's model the probability of relapse is significantly affected by individuals' perception of their ability to successfully cope with high risk situations. People are most likely to avoid relapse if (1) they can identify and anticipate high risk situations and (2) they have confidence in the coping skills they have available to deal with the situation. Annis' research produced two clinical assessment instruments that provide another example of individual variability among substance abusers. The Inventory of Drinking Situations (IDS) shows that individuals differ in terms of the situations that pose a high relapse risk. The Situational Confidence Questionnaire (SCQ) demonstrates individual differences in perceived confidence to handle various classes of situations. Knowledge of a client's IDS and SCQ profiles enables the counselor to develop relapse prevention plans that address each client's individual strengths and weaknesses.

Summary: The Homogeneity Assumption

Controlled research does not support the assertion that alcoholics and addicts form a homogeneous group who have a unitary disease caused solely by a genetic defect. To the contrary, it appears that there is great individual variability among people labeled as alcoholics or addicts. Recent research suggests that there are individual differences in the sequence of events experienced by substance abusers rather than a predictable path or progression. It highlights differences in drug-related behavior, expectancies, and readiness to change rather than common personality traits.

If alcoholics and addicts do not form a homogeneous group, then it seems unlikely that a standard core treatment will meet their diverse needs. The next section addresses the question of treatment effectiveness: Is traditional treatment the most effective approach?

The "Does It Work?" Question

Some clinicians have been encouraged in their training to identify the superior therapeutic approach and adopt it to the exclusion of all others. Treatment models tend to be categorized as works and doesn't work, with outcome research interpreted as proving that an intervention is or is not effective. This dichotomous good approach/ bad approach mentality seems particularly prevalent among substance abuse treatment professionals.

Is traditional substance abuse treatment effective? The complexity of this seemingly simple question has been discussed at length in numerous reviews (e.g., Baekeland, Lundwall, & Kissin, 1975; Institute of Medicine, 1990; Miller & Hester, 1986a; Saxe, Dougherty, Esty, & Fine, 1983). Nathan and Skinstad (1987) have noted that much of the research is fraught with major methodological weaknesses that render it uninterpretable. For example, it has been difficult to determine the effectiveness of Alcoholics Anonymous because most of the research is poorly controlled. Saxe, Dougherty, Esty, and Fine (1983) note that it is impossible to distinguish whether the reputed success of AA is attributable to the Twelve Steps or to selection bias. That is, if the most motivated persons with the best prognosis join and comply with AA, is the positive outcome due to AA or to the prior characteristics of the subjects? Would the most motivated subjects with the best prognosis have improved regardless of the intervention they received– psychotherapy, a support group not based on the Twelve Steps, or even a placebo drug treatment? These questions cannot be answered unless subject selection bias is explicitly controlled by the research design.

Miller and Hester (1986a), in their exhaustive review of controlled research, found that the techniques most commonly employed in traditional treatment programs were *not* supported by controlled research. Ironically, the procedures that *are* supported by controlled research (primarily the behavioral interventions) tend to be ignored by most traditional programs (Miller, 1987).

What can we conclude from this research? First, there is *not* overwhelming support for the effectiveness of traditional treatment. While uncontrolled anecdotal sources sometimes claim remarkably high success rates (see Emrick & Hansen, 1983), controlled outcome studies seldom report success rates exceeding 30 to 50%. The research clearly does not justify claims of proven effectiveness nor the proclamation that traditional treatment is the best or only way to treat addictions. Furthermore, the recent Institute of Medicine (1990) report expresses concerns that some treatment approaches, particularly those that ignore individual differences and impose a treatment philosophy through negative confrontation, may actually *harm* the patient. The Institute claims that "some people with alcohol problems are made worse by treatment" (p. 157).

While the evidence from controlled research contrasts with the one best way assumption, it should not be interpreted as a blanket indictment of traditional treatment. The old saying about the gas tank being half full or half empty applies here; while a 30 to 50% success rate is hardly overwhelming, it indicates that a substantial number of people apparently *do* get better in traditional treatment.

Nonetheless, this partial success should not obscure the fact that there is room for improvement. Miller and Hester (1986a) note that a significant number of procedures which have a strong research base are underutilized. Miller (1987) argues that this is due to treatment programs' reluctance to adopt procedures which are not part of the established routine of traditional treatment. There are empirically-tested treatment approaches that might succeed where the traditional approach does not, but newer approaches are often ignored by treatment providers.

Does traditional treatment work? There is a simple answer to this complex question: It works for some people, but it clearly does not work for others. Miller and Hester (1986b) found that a treatment procedure is most likely to be effective when it addresses a specific deficit in the individual client. Miller and Hester, along with Marlatt (1988), Nathan (1986) and the Institute of Medicine (1990) have interpreted this research to support the *matching hypothesis*. Contrary to the one best way assumption, research suggests that prescriptive services, using empirically-tested procedures targeted to individual client needs, are more likely to be effective than the standard core treatment protocol.

Motivation and Denial

The matching hypothesis has important implications for the issues of denial, motivation to change, and adherence to treatment. Historically, denial and resistance to change have been interpreted as symptoms of addiction. Treatment programs have absolved themselves of any responsibility for treatment failures by explaining that they cannot be expected to help uncooperative clients who may need to hit bottom. However, it is equally plausible that denial and resistance are *induced by treatment*: When clients are offered one and only one treatment approach, and that approach is not matched to their individual characteristics and needs, resistance is not necessarily a sign of pathological denial. Perhaps denial is more a reflection of limited treatment options and lack of individualization rather than an inevitable symptom of addiction. Miller (1985) offers an in-depth analysis of this alternative view of motivation and denial and describes a non-confrontational motivational interview approach (Miller, 1989) that can elicit client concern and cooperation while minimizing resistance.

In summary, evidence from controlled research does not support the validity of any single treatment model. Alcoholics and addicts do not form a homogeneous group, and the standard core treatment has not been proven to meet their diverse needs. While it is clear that many people get better through the traditional approach, it is just as clear that many others need a different approach.

SUBSTANCE ABUSE TREATMENT:
WHERE WE ARE GOING

There are several movements which are converging to promote a shift in how substance abuse treatment services are provided. First, more graduate-trained clinicians are becoming involved in substance abuse treatment. Many tend to question clinical dogma and look to the scientific literature for empirically-tested treatment procedures and approaches. As the field moves from a craft to a professional orientation, more clinicians are becoming aware of the limitations of the one best way assumption and recognizing the need for genuinely individualized treatment. Insurance companies and corporate health benefits managers are carefully reviewing the outcome literature and becoming increasingly unwilling to fund expensive treatment that fails to help the majority of clients. This section will describe where the field is going and how rehabilitation professionals can use this information to help their clients gain access to individualized and effective treatment.

There is encouraging evidence that the substance abuse treatment field is moving *from dogmatic argumentation to client-centered individualized treatment.* Unfortunately, our propensity to declare treatment approaches good or bad has created an adversarial atmosphere; proponents of an approach defend their model from what they perceive as attacks by those who cite disconfirming research. While there is no question that millions of people believe that AA helped them recover, it is also clear that controlled research does not support the effectiveness of AA (Miller & Hester, 1986a,b). This can be interpreted as an attack on AA or as an indication that AA helps some people but does not help others.

The adversarial atmosphere and the good approach/bad approach mind set have clouded the real question: Which approach works best for whom under what conditions? Rather than declaring Twelve-Step interventions good or bad, we should attempt to differentially assess those who are or are not likely to comply with and benefit from that approach. Rather than defending procedures, we should attempt to *expand* our repertoire of clinical tools, to serve those who benefit from traditional treatment as well as those who need other approaches. Rather than forcing people to fit a predetermined program that does not match their characteristics, we should design a program to fit the individual, prescriptively matching procedures and approaches to client needs.

The substance abuse treatment field seems to be moving *from an ideology-driven craft to a scientifically-based* professional discipline. Rather than using theoretical constructs such as denial to rationalize treatment failures, we are finally looking to the literature for tested procedures and approaches that are more effective in helping people comply with and benefit from treatment. While there is no question that firsthand experience is invaluable, recovering counselors need to recognize that different people need different paths to sobriety. They will be most effective if they can open their minds to empirically-validated treatment alternatives, especially to those approaches which differ from the way that worked for them.

Controlled research results clearly lend more support to the matching hypothesis than to the homogeneity assumption. Consequently, substance abuse assessments should move *from binary diagnostic labeling to multidimensional functional assessments.* A comprehensive assessment should address alcohol and other drug use, problems in other life areas that are caused by substance abuse, and problems in other life areas that contribute to substance abuse. This contrasts with a narrow drug-centered assessment which assumes that substance abuse is always the primary problem. The assessment should be differentiating rather than pigeonholing, describing the distinguishing characteristics of a unique person instead of trying to funnel a heterogeneous group of people into diagnostic categories. Rather than attempting to distinguish alcoholics from nonalcoholics, our assessments should focus on differences among people who abuse drugs and how those differences can be used to develop an individualized and prescriptive treatment plan. The most valuable assessment will have clear implications for differentiated treatment, explicitly pointing out the links between the situation and characteristics of the individual client and specific treatment recommendations. It should show the logical relationship between the assessment results and the treatment recommendations, with specific problems or deficits addressed by specific therapeutic strategies, rather than assuming that the diagnostic label dictates the treatment.

IMPLICATIONS FOR THE REFERRING PROFESSIONAL

There are several steps that the rehabilitation professional can take to become more effective in referring clients to individualized treatment that is most appropriately matched to their individual characteristics and needs. Most important, the referring professional must be well informed about substance abuse treatment, with the background knowledge necessary to engage in a meaningful dialogue with treatment providers. Many treatment programs are steadfastly committed to the one best way assumption, and will be reluctant to provide treatment that differs from their usual mode of operation. The referring professional will need to be able to identify treatment programs that are willing and able to provide individualized treatment for their clients. Chapter 16 provides detailed and specific guidelines for the referring professional, including arranging assessments, evaluating individual treatment programs, and case management and client advocacy. The information contained in Hester's chapter of this volume will also be helpful.

Professionals who refer clients to treatment are in a unique position to select treatment providers who provide innovative research-based interventions that meet the needs of their clients. The referring professional can encourage treatment programs to provide functional behavioral assessments and demand genuinely individualized treatment protocols. By insisting on differentiating assessments and differentiated treatment, referring professionals can help ensure that their clients receive treatment appropriately matched to their needs.

Disability Issues

Once appropriate treatment providers have been identified, rehabilitation professionals can work with them to accommodate the needs of persons with disabilities. Specific issues and strategies for each of the four steps in this process are discussed in more detail in Chapter 16.

The first step is to promote treatment programs' interest in and commitment to services for persons with a dual disability. Treatment programs will carefully assess the need for new services and will attempt to ensure that there is a reasonable expectation of sufficient referrals to support a program. Chapter 16 also discusses alternative strategies for situations where substance abuse treatment providers are not willing or able to accommodate persons with other disabilities.

After a commitment to dual disability services is secured, those in the rehabilitation sector will need to help treatment programs understand and deal with basic disability issues. This includes areas such as staff sensitivity to the concerns of persons with disabilities, accessibility, nursing needs, adaptive equipment, and communication alternatives.

The third step is to anticipate and avoid specific problems that might arise between the rehabilitation and substance abuse sectors. Conflicts over the use of prescription medication by persons in recovery is one example.

The final step is the ongoing process of maintaining dialogue and communication links among all involved in rehabilitation and treatment efforts. Frequent personal interaction will be a key to ensuring that the different sectors work together through coordinated services that address the needs and goals of each individual.

REFERENCES

Alcoholics Anonymous World Services (1976). Alcoholics Anonymous. New York: Author.

Annis, H.A., & Davis, C.S. (1989). Relapse prevention. In R.K. Hester & W.R. Miller (Eds.), *Handbook of alcoholism treatment approaches: Effective alternatives* (pp. 170-182). New York: Pergamon.

Baekeland, F., Lundwall, L., & Kissin, B. (1975). Methods for the treatment of chronic alcoholism: A critical appraisal. In R. Gibbons et al. (Eds.) *Research advances in alcohol and drug problems.* New York: Wiley.

Blane, H.T., & Leonard, K.E. (1987). *Psychological theories of drinking and alcoholism.* New York: Guilford.

Blum, K. et al. (1990). Allelic association of human dopamine D2 receptor gene in alcoholism. *Journal of the American Medical Association, 263*(15), 2055-2060.

Blume, S. (1983). *The disease concept today.* Minneapolis: The Johnson Institute.

Bohman, M., Cloninger, C., von Knorring, A., & Sigvardsson, S. (1984). An adoption study of somatoform disorders. III. Cross-fostering analysis and genetic relationship to alcoholism and criminality. *Archives of General Psychiatry, 41,* 872-878.

Cahalan, D., & Room, R. (1974). *Problem drinking among American men.* New Brunswick, NJ: Rutgers Center of Alcohol Studies.

Clark, W., & Cahalan, D. (1976). Changes in problem drinking over a four-year span. *Addictive Behaviors, 1,* 251-259.

Cloninger, C. (1983). Genetic and environmental factors in the development of alcoholism. *Journal of Psychiatric Treatment and Evaluation, 5,* 487-496.

Cox, M. (1987). Personality theory and research. In H.T. Blane & K.E. Leonard (Eds.), *Psychological theories of drinking and alcoholism* (pp. 55-89). New York: Guilford.

Emrick, C.D., & Hansen, J. (1983). Assertions regarding effectiveness of treatment for alcoholism. *American Psychologist, 38,* 1078-1088.

Fillmore, K. (1975). Relationships between specific drinking problems in early adulthood and middle age: An exploratory 20-year follow-up study. *Journal of Studies on Alcohol, 36,* 882-907.

Fillmore, K., & Midanik, L. (1984). Chronicity of drinking problems among men: A longitudinal study. *Journal of Studies on Alcohol, 45,* 228-236.

Filstead, W. (1984). Levels of care for alcoholism and substance abuse: A conceptual framework for organizing and delivering treatment services. In M.J. Goby (Ed.), *Alcoholism: Treatment and recovery* (pp. 49-57). St. Louis: Catholic Health Association of the United States.

Fingarette, H. (1988). *Heavy drinking: The myth of alcoholism as a disease.* Berkeley: University of California Press.

Glatt, M. (1958). Group therapy in alcoholism. *British Journal of Addiction, 54,* 133-138.

Goodwin, D.W. (1988). *Is alcoholism hereditary?* New York: Ballantine Books.

Goodwin, D., Schulsinger, F., Hermansen, L., Guze, S., & Winokur, G. (1973). Alcohol problems in adoptees raised apart from alcoholic biological parents. *Archives of General Psychiatry, 28,* 238-243.

Goodwin, D., Schulsinger, F., Moller, N., Hermansen, L., Winokur, G., & Guze, S. (1974). Drinking problems in adopted and nonadopted sons of alcoholics. *Archives of General Psychiatry, 31,* 164-169.

Graham, J., & Strenger, V. (1988). MMPI characteristics of alcoholics: A review. *Journal of Consulting and Clinical Psychology, 56,* 197-205.

Horn, J.L., Wanberg, K.W., & Foster, F.M. (1987). *Guide to the alcohol use inventory.* Minneapolis: National Computer Systems.

Institute of Medicine. (1990). *Broadening the base of treatment for alcohol problems.* Washington, DC: National Academy Press.

Jellinek, E.M. (1946). Phases in the drinking history of alcoholics. *Quarterly Journal of Studies on Alcohol, 7,* 1-88.

Jellinek, E.M. (1952). Phases of alcohol addiction. *Quarterly Journal of Studies on Alcohol, 13,* 673-684.

Jellinek, E.M. (1960). *The disease concept of alcoholism.* New Brunswick, NJ: College and University Press. (Out of print; reprints available from National Council on Alcoholism, New York, NY).

Johnson, V.E. (1980). *I'll quit tomorrow.* New York: Harper & Row.

Marlatt, G.A. (1988). Matching clients to treatment: Treatment models and stages of change. In D.M. Donovan & G.A. Marlatt (Eds.), *Assessment of addictive behaviors* (pp. 474-483). New York: Guilford.

Marlatt, G.A., & Gordon, J.R. (1985). *Relapse prevention.* New York: Guilford.

Miller, W.R. (1985). Motivation for treatment: A review with special emphasis on alcoholism. *Psychological Bulletin, 98,* 84-107.

Miller, W.R. (1987). Behavioral alcohol treatment research advances: Barriers to utilization. *Advances in Behavior Research & Therapy, 9,* 145-164.

Miller, W.R. (1989). Increasing motivation for change. In R.K. Hester & W.R. Miller (Eds.), *Handbook of alcoholism treatment approaches: Effective alternatives* (pp. 67-80). New York: Pergamon.

Miller, W.R., & Hester, R.K. (1986a). The effectiveness of alcoholism treatment: What research reveals. In W.R. Miller & N. Heather (Eds.), *Treating addictive behaviors: Processes of change* (pp. 121-174). New York: Plenum.

Miller, W.R., & Hester, R.K. (1986b). Matching problem drinkers with optimal treatments. In W.R. Miller & N. Heather (Eds.), *Treating addictive behaviors: Processes of change* (pp. 175-204). New York: Plenum.

Mueller, L., & Ketcham, K. (1987). *Recovering: How to get and stay sober.* New York: Bantam.

Mulford, H. (1984). Rethinking the alcohol problem: A natural processes model. *Journal of Drug Issues, 14,* 31-43.

Nathan, P.E. (1986). What do behavioral scientists know–and what can they do–about alcoholism. In P.C. Clayton (Ed.), *Nebraska symposium on motivation: Alcohol and addictive behavior* (pp. 1-26). Lincoln: University of Nebraska Press.

Nathan, P. E. (1988). The addictive personality is the behavior of the addict. *Journal of Consulting and Clinical Psychology, 56,* 183-188.

Nathan, P.E., & Skinstad, A. (1987). Outcomes of treatment for alcohol problems: Current methods, problems, and results. *Journal of Consulting and Clinical Psychology, 55,* 332-340.

Pattison, E., Sobell, M., & Sobell, L. (1977). *Emerging concepts of alcohol dependence.* New York: Springer.

Polich, J., Armor, D., & Braiker, H. (1981). *The course of alcoholism: Four years after treatment.* New York: Wiley.

Prochaska, J., & DiClemente, C. (1986). Towards a comprehensive model of change. In W.R. Miller & N. Heather (Eds.), *Treating addictive behaviors: Processes of change* (pp. 3-28). New York: Plenum.

Saxe, L., Dougherty, D., Esty, K., & Fine, M. (1983). *The effectiveness and costs of alcoholism treatment.* Health Technology Case Study 22. Washington, DC: Office of Technology Assessment.

Schuckit, M. (1987). Biological vulnerability to alcoholism. *Journal of Consulting and Clinical Psychology, 55,* 301-309.

Selzer, M. (1971). The Michigan alcoholism screening test: The quest for a new diagnostic instrument. *American Journal of Psychiatry, 127,* 1653-1658.

Skinner, H. (1982). Statistical approaches to the classification of alcohol and drug addiction. *British Journal of Addiction*, *77*, 259-273.

Sutker, P., & Allain, A. (1988). Issues in personality conceptualizations of addictive behaviors. *Journal of Consulting and Clinical Psychology*, *56*, 172-182.

Vaillant, G.E. (1983). *The natural history of alcoholism*. Cambridge, MA: Harvard University.

von Knorring, L., von Knorring, A., Smigan, L., Lindberg, U., & Edholm, M. (1987). Personality traits in subtypes of alcoholics. *Journal of Studies on Alcohol*, *48*(6), 523-527.

Wilsnack, R., Wilsnack, S., & Klassen, A. (1986). Antecedents and consequences of drinking and drinking problems in women: Patterns from a U.S. national survey. In P.C. Clayton (Ed.), *Nebraska symposium on motivation: Alcohol and addictive behavior* (pp. 85-158). Lincoln: University of Nebraska Press.

Zucker, R.A. (1986). The four alcoholisms: A developmental account of the etiologic process. In P.C. Clayton (Ed.), *Nebraska symposium on motivation: Alcohol and addictive behavior* (pp. 27-84). Lincoln: University of Nebraska Press.

Chapter 10

Clinical Features of Traditional Chemical Dependence Treatment Programs in the United States

Martin Doot, MD

Understanding the beginnings of the traditional treatment model for alcohol and drug dependence in the United States is enhanced by a brief historical overview. I use the term Traditional treatment model for lack of an accepted label to describe these programs. An alternate label is the 28-day treatment program. In these days of cost containment and shorter lengths of hospital stays, the label could be easily misunderstood. Treatment programs in the United States have resisted assuming the label of the Minnesota Model used more prominently in the foreign medical literature. However, the best review of this model was published under that title by Cook in the *British Journal of Addiction* in 1988.

The origins of the model can be clearly traced to the collaboration of professionals from a number of disciplines with recovering alcoholics in Alcoholics Anonymous (AA). AA was started by two alcoholics in 1935. It remains a spiritual program of recovery based on 12 steps developed as a self-help group open to anyone with a desire to stop drinking. By tradition, the names of the recovering alcoholics who collaborated with the professionals often remain anonymous. The strength of the AA principles and the personal recoveries of these early AA members, however, is what strongly influenced the professionals who helped develop the model.

The professionals who worked with two of the three programs mentioned in Cook's article all started working at the same facility. Nelson J. Bradley and Dan Anderson were a staff physician and psychology student working at Hastings State Hospital with Dr. Ralph Rossen, superintendent of the hospital, and Fred E., a recovering alcoholic who was Dr. Rossen's administrative assistant. Dr. Rossen later became commissioner of Mental Health in Minnesota and appointed Dr. Bradley as superintendent of the Willmar State Hospital in Willmar, Minnesota. He asked Dr. Anderson, Fred E. and a number of other recovering alcoholics to join him in developing a program for the chronic alcoholics who were admitted to the state hospital. At the time, their services included detoxification and custodial care for the individuals who had chronic organic brain syndrome and could not return to their communities. These original professionals were later joined by Dr. Jean Rossi, a clinical psychologist, and John Keller, a Lutheran pastor. Dr. Anderson left to help develop what is today Hazelden treatment programs. Drs. Bradley and Rossi and John Keller were invited to develop the alcoholism program at Lutheran General Hospital in Park Ridge, Illinois, which has developed Parkside Medical Services Corporation, a network of treatment programs across the United States and in Sweden. Both programs developed counselor training programs which provide addiction counselors and administrative personnel for many programs across the country.

Table 1 lists the 12 steps of AA. These steps have been adapted by other 12-step recovery programs which have developed specifically for persons with other drug dependencies and compulsive disorders. The professional treatment program was developed to provide a variety of treatment experiences which were carefully designed to foster sustained sobriety together with lifestyle changes which would prevent relapse and improve the quality of living and relationships. The changes often mean changes in risky behavior, avoiding people, places and things associated with drug use, learning a lifestyle of honesty, and asking for help from others, rather than one of manipulation and self-reliance.

ASSESSMENT

Active alcoholic or drug dependent patients can bring with them a host of medical, psychiatric, psychosocial and spiritual difficulties which are revealed during an initial assessment. Issues addressed

TABLE 1. The Twelve Steps of Alcoholics Anonymous

Step 1.   We admitted we were powerless over alcohol–that our lives had become unmanageable.

Step 2.   Came to believe that a power greater than ourselves could restore us to sanity.

Step 3.   Made a decision to turn our Will and lives over to the care of God as we understood Him.

Step 4.   Made a searching and fearless inventory of ourselves.

Step 5.   Admitted to God, and to ourselves, and to another human being the exact nature of our wrongs.

Step 6.   Were entirely ready to have God remove all these defects of character.

Step 7.   Humbly asked Him to remove our shortcomings.

Step 8.   Made a list of all persons we had harmed and became willing to make amends to them all.

Step 9.   Made direct amends to such people wherever possible, except when to do so would injure them or others.

Step 10.   Continued to take personal inventory and when we were wrong promptly admitted it.

Step 11.   Sought through prayer and meditation to improve our conscious contact with God as we understood Him, praying only for knowledge of this will for us and the power to carry that out.

Step 12.   Having had a spiritual awakening as a result of these steps, we tried to carry this message to other alcoholics and practice these principles in all our affairs.

during the assessments, completed by the members of the staff of the treatment program, include the following:

1. Acute intoxication and management of withdrawal.
2. Physical complications and concurrent physical illness.
3. Psychiatric complications and concurrent psychiatric illness.
4. Life area impairments.
5. Treatment acceptance or resistance.

6. Loss of control or relapse potential.
7. Recovery environment.

The assessment of these issues is accomplished by a staff of professionals from a variety of backgrounds. A traditional program will include the following staff and their roles:

A *physician* is responsible for the history and physical examination, mental status examination, differential diagnosis, assuring a safe detoxification, treatment of medical and psychiatric complications and concurrent illness, and monitoring of the progress of rehabilitation.

Nursing staff provide the nursing assessment, nursing care plans, and 24-hour nursing care during detoxification and in rehabilitation settings where patients need that level of intensity for medical and psychiatric illness.

Addiction counselors are responsible for the alcohol and drug assessment as well as a psychosocial and spiritual assessment. They provide individual counseling and group therapy with a specific addiction focus.

Recreation therapists are responsible for an assessment of leisure activities and provide counseling and new experiences in treatment dealing with leisure time.

Family counselors and therapists are responsible for the assessment of the family of addicted patients and provide family and group therapy for these families.

A *clinical psychologist* provides psychological assessments and psychological testing and is used by the counselors as a consultant for help in individual counseling and group therapy.

Available to the core staff of a traditional program are a variety of *consultants* to meet specific patient needs. Addiction counselors may come from a variety of professional or recovery backgrounds. *Social workers* and *clergy* may work as consulting professionals or as addiction counselors.

MODEL PHILOSOPHY

The unique nature of the program is not the group of professionals (with the exception of the recovering addiction counselor). A similar staff would be available in a psychiatric unit. What makes them unique is how they use the assessment data and their treatment skills, and how they work together. The model philosophy described by Cook (1988) defines the unique nature of these programs. These beliefs include:

1. The possibility that addicted individuals and their families can change their beliefs, attitudes and behaviors.
2. The disease concept which focuses the patient on the addiction as the primary problem, not as a symptom of another problem.
3. Treatment goals of abstinence from all mood-altering chemicals and improvement of lifestyle.
4. The principles of AA and the other 12-step programs.

PROGRAM ELEMENTS AND STRUCTURE

The major focus of program activities and individual counseling with the patients is directed at ameliorating their lack of knowledge, confronting their psychological defenses, and revealing the enabling systems which keep the addicted individuals and their families from accepting their illness and making the appropriate lifestyle changes to maintain a life of abstinence and spiritual growth.

The program elements and structure include the following:

1. *Group therapy:* The place where the defenses that maintain denial and block the feelings associated with the unmanageable life are confronted by peers and counselor.
2. *Lectures:* Where education about the disease and recovery issues are presented and then processed.
3. *Individual counseling:* Done by addiction counselors, many of whom are recovering themselves.
4. *Family counseling:* Education, group and individual counseling, and motivation to use self-help groups.
5. *Goal-oriented assignments:* Often processed in the peer groups.
6. *Therapeutic community:* An environment which emphasizes acceptance of the need for abstinence with the limitations

associated with it, but responsibility in other life areas. Admitting powerlessness is not learned helplessness, but rather learning to live and cope responsibly without the use of addicting chemicals.

7. *Multidisciplinary assessment:* Used to develop a master treatment plan that is focused on the primary problems of addiction and which avoids defocusing on problems which have the potential for resolution with abstinence and a recovery program.

8. *Recreation therapy:* Focused on building self-esteem and finding alternatives to the time spent using chemicals.

9. *Twelve-step orientation:* Done by the counselors in groups, lectures and in individual sessions, and by volunteers from 12-step programs. All staff look for opportunities to teach the use of recovery tools in the treatment process. They will look for opportunities to help patients practice honest sharing, resolving conflicts, trusting others, and asking for help.

10. *Twelve-step program:* Involvement includes AA or other meetings in the treatment facility and in the patient's community with peer and staff processing after the experience.

Patients are admitted to the program and are expected to participate in all of the core treatment activities according to a structured schedule designed to keep them focused on the problem of addiction and recovery. Patients are not offered a cure for their addiction, but rather the tools to live free of compulsive use with the help of others and a spiritual program of recovery. The staff's expectation is the need for professional help until the patient and family can use a self-help, 12-step group for continued recovery. These structured services are provided at various intensities in what is known as levels of care:

Level 1: Mutual self-help, 12-step program.

Level 2: Low intensity (1 session per week) outpatient. This service is called continuing care when it is provided after a more intensive primary treatment.

Level 3: Intensive outpatient, 3 to 4 sessions per week for 4 to 6 weeks.

Level 4: Intensive day hospital, 5 to 7 days per week of day programming.

Level 5: Residential treatment.

Level 6: Specialty hospital or acute care hospital unit.

Outcome studies of patients in this model were begun as early as 1955 with patients treated at Willmar State Hospital. In addition to the studies cited by Cook (1988), the research staff of Parkside Medical Services have continued to document program success. In spite of the methodological problems of patient selection, nonrandomization, difficulties with finding adequate control groups, and questions of validity of self and significant other reports, some conclusions are consistent enough to be impressive. When the total treatment group is included, nearly 45% recovery or improvement is demonstrated (Cook, 1988). When patients complete the course of primary treatment and continuing care and remain involved in a 12-step group, more than two-thirds of the patients maintain stable recoveries (Cross, 1990). The follow-up of 1987 admissions to Parkside residential treatment programs and 1988 inpatient, residential and outpatient programs demonstrated similar results (Filstead, 1989, 1990).

The traditional model of treatment has been adapted from the original model at Willmar State Hospital to deal with other drug addictions and special patient populations, but its flexibility has limitations. The limitations may relate to: (1) Program philosophy, (2) staff skills, (3) program elements, (4) therapeutic community, (5) program schedule, (6) the facility, and (7) 12-step groups.

PATIENTS WITH DUAL DISABILITIES

Problems with the model when it was modified to assist patients with dual psychiatric and substance abuse diagnoses are listed below:

1. The program philosophy of abstinence from all mood altering chemicals and focus on symptoms as complications of the addiction has led to the inappropriate termination or withhold-

ing of psychotropic medications for patients with affective disorders or psychotic illness.
2. Lack of staff skills with psychiatric populations can lead to inaccurate diagnosis, inappropriate or insufficient treatment, and inability to focus the patient on treatment tasks.
3. The program may lack patient education about psychiatric illness and medications.
4. Confrontive addiction-focused group therapy may not be tolerated.
5. The therapeutic community may not accept this *different* patient. The patient may not identify with the problems of the peers and use this as a defense to avoid accepting their illness.
6. The fast pace of the schedule may not be tolerated.
7. The facility may not be designed to protect suicidal patients.
8. Twelve-step group members may not accept someone on medication.

PROGRAM MODIFICATIONS FOR PATIENTS WITH DUAL DIAGNOSES

The dual diagnosis unit at Parkside Lutheran Hospital has struggled successfully with these limitations by making several modifications of the traditional program.

1. Abstinence means avoiding medications with addiction potential. Education is provided to patients individually and in groups by physicians and nurses and reinforced by counselors to take appropriate psychotropic medications for concurrent illness.
2. The psychiatrist on the team has years of experience in differential diagnoses and treatment. He is board-certified in psychiatry and certified in addiction medicine. The nursing staff has psychiatric and addiction experience. The counselors are trained in dual diagnosis and the psychologist provides additional input.
3. The program schedule includes dual diagnosis and medication groups as well as addiction groups.

4. Patients are evaluated and referred to the unit from other Parkside programs. Patients not needing the specialized services are encouraged to seek treatment at a residential level with a traditional program.
5. The schedule is individualized; an inability to meet the schedule demands is assessed carefully before it is confronted.
6. The facility would ideally be on a locked unit. Suicidal patients are still transferred to a locked unit until they are stable. Continuity of care is maintained by substance abuse staff on the psychiatric unit.
7. Volunteers and staff provide educational lectures to the AA community. A new 12-step group was started: MIRA (Mentally Ill Recovering Alcoholics). These groups provide an understanding place to talk about psychiatric symptoms and medication while in recovery from alcoholism.

CHEMICAL DEPENDENCE TREATMENT FOR PERSONS WITH PHYSICAL DISABILITIES

The Minnesota Model has also been modified for persons with physical disabilities who have substance abuse problems. Parkside has recently collaborated in a pilot program with American Rehabilitation Centers in the development of an addiction treatment program for persons with physical impairments. The limitations in the treatment model it must overcome are:

1. The philosophy of powerlessness over the drugs of abuse must not be extended to a sense of helplessness and hopelessness related to the physical disability.
2. Special staff skills must be developed that relate to the assessment and care of persons with physical disabilities.
3. Patients with impaired cognitive abilities resulting from head trauma are accommodated so as to minimize interference with the educational parts of the program.
4. A therapeutic community is difficult to nurture without peers who have similar physical needs.

5. The addiction treatment schedule must provide time for physical therapies.
6. Facilities must be made accessible to persons with physical disabilities.
7. Access must be provided to self-help, 12-step groups despite physical and attitudinal barriers.

PROGRAM MODIFICATIONS FOR PATIENTS WITH PHYSICAL DISABILITIES

The pilot program has addressed these potential limitations by:

1. Verbalizing the philosophy of treatment to enhance patients assuming responsibility for continuing their physical rehabilitation during treatment for addiction.
2. Including additional staff such as nurse's aides, a rehabilitation nurse provided by the rehabilitation company to guide the rehabilitation care plans, physical and occupational therapists, and physiatrist and neuropsychologist as consultants.
3. Including within the program treatment modalities which are needed for persons with physical disabilities.
4. A peer group of addicted patients with physical disabilities can be established by referral from other substance abuse programs and rehabilitation units.
5. Modifying the schedule to fit the physical rehabilitation and addictions program components together.
6. Making the facility and 12-step meeting fully accessible.

A brief case history illustrates how a traditional addictions program was modified to serve an individual with a physical disability. R.T. was a young man who sustained a cervical spine injury while intoxicated. He left the rehabilitation unit at the acute care hospital against medical advice before completing physical rehabilitation in order to drink. He was later admitted to an alcohol rehabilitation unit for detoxification and treatment of his addiction. He was the only patient with a physical disability on the unit at the time and left before completing treatment. He was readmitted to the alcohol unit within 9 months. After detoxification he was transferred to the pilot program for persons with disabilities who also have addictions. He was in treatment with four other patients who had physical disabilities. His needs were met by the specially trained staff which allowed him to finish the program with improvement in both areas of his needs. His case illustrates how successful treatment of an addiction is enhanced by modifying a traditional program.

The traditional model of treatment has developed to address the most common needs of alcohol and drug dependent patients and their families. This model of treatment can be adapted to meet the needs of special populations including persons with physical disabilities. Careful planning necessitates examination of program philosophy, staff skills, therapeutic modalities, schedule, facilities and interaction with 12-step groups. Programs focusing on these special needs should be developed regionally with referral from both addictions and physical rehabilitation units.

REFERENCES

Cook, D.D. (1988). The Minnesota model and the management of drug and alcohol dependency: Miracle, method, or myth? *British Journal of Addiction*, *83*(6), 625- 634, *83*(7) 735-748.

Cross, Gerald M. (1990). Alcoholism treatment: A ten-year follow-up study. *Alcoholism: Clinical and Experimental Research*, *14*, 169-173.

Filstead, W.J. (1989). Treatment outcome: An evaluation of adult residential treatment services. Parkside Medical Services Corporation.

Filstead, W.J. (1990). Treatment outcome: An evaluation of adult and youth treatment services. Parkside Medical Services Corporation.

Parkside Medical Services Corporation. (1989). *Standards of Care, Addiction Services*.

Chapter 11

Matching Clients to Alcohol Treatments: What Little We Know and How Very Far We Have to Go

Reid K. Hester, PhD

Eleven years ago, in the fall of 1978, Bill Miller and I met as I began my internship in clinical psychology. While discussing various projects we might collaborate on, we agreed that the field of alcoholism treatment research was growing by leaps and bounds and was in need of a comprehensive and critical review of the literature. To be truly comprehensive we agreed to review all of the treatment outcome studies we could find in languages we could understand. We had no idea what lay in store for us. Six months later we completed our review of more than 600 studies and began to write the chapter which summarized our findings (Miller & Hester, 1980).

Completing this review and surveying the results left us with mixed emotions. First, we were amazed at the sheer size of the literature and the number of different types of treatments which had been tried with alcoholics and alcohol abusers. Second, a common pattern seemed to emerge for many treatments which have fallen into disuse. Initial, uncontrolled studies would report impressive and exciting outcomes only to have later, more methodologically rigorous and controlled studies find little or no specific benefit from the same treatment. On the other hand, there were a number of alternative treatments which received consistent support from controlled research. This reinforced to us the value of systematic, controlled and comparative research. It was difficult to come to any firm conclusions about the effectiveness of a number of the treatment approaches in this review because the picture was so muddled with the results of uncontrolled studies which often had significant confounds.

Late in 1983 we decided to update our original review. This time, however, we only included treatment outcome studies which had either control groups, comparison groups, or some sort of matched group. This decision to exclude uncontrolled studies resulted in a much clearer picture of the effectiveness of alcoholism treatment approaches. Our findings were encouraging but also disconcerting. First, it became clear that there is no one treatment approach which is effective for all alcohol abusers. The answer, so long sought after, does not exist. Instead, there are a number of alternative interventions. Second, these alternative interventions are consistently supported by controlled research. What was disconcerting was our realization that none of these interventions was commonly used in alcoholism treatment programs in the United States. Even more distressing, we found that none of the common elements of alcoholism treatment in the United States are supported by controlled research. There was virtually no overlap between what treatments are supported by research and what treatments are in common use in the United States. Table 1 lists the bottom line conclusions of our second literature review (Miller & Hester, 1986a).

TABLE 1. Supported versus Standard Alcoholism Treatment Methods

Treatment methods currently supported by controlled outcome research	Treatment methods currently employed as standard practice in alcoholism programs
Aversion therapies	Alcoholics Anonymous
Behavioral Self-Control Training	Alcoholism education
Community Reinforcement Approach	Confrontation
Marital and Family therapy	Disulfiram
Social skills training	Group therapy
Stress management	Individual counseling

Reprinted with permission from W. R. Miller & N. Heather (Eds.), *Treating Addictive Behaviors: Processes of Change.* New York: Plenum.

This second review of the literature led us to discover a number of controlled studies of the relative effectiveness of the setting, length, and intensity of treatment. So naturally we decided to write yet another review focusing specifically on these studies (Miller & Hester, 1986b). Again, somewhat to our amazement, the 24 controlled studies were consistent in their findings. None of these studies found any significant differences in outcome measures at follow-up when patients were randomly assigned to receive either shorter vs. longer treatment, more intense vs. less intense treatment, inpatient or outpatient treatment. In fact, the trends which existed favored shorter and less intensive treatment settings. Several researchers, however, did note that patients with greater social instability and/or greater problem severity seemed to differentially benefit from more intensive or longer treatment. Needless to say, this created something of a stir in the alcoholism field. In any event, the results of this review suggested to us that it is the content of treatment which is important, not the setting in which it occurs.

While sifting through all these articles, we also came across a number of reports of significant interactions between client characteristics and treatments which influenced outcomes. Figure 1 illustrates a simple hypothetical client-treatment interaction and how it can substantially influence outcome. For example, one client characteristic could be conceptual level ranging from concrete to abstract. Clients with low conceptual abilities have a better outcome with treatment B than with treatment A, while the opposite is true for clients with high levels of conceptual abilities. In actuality, McLachlan (1974) did find such an interaction between clients' conceptual level and the therapists' conceptual level. When the two matched, outcome was significantly better than when there was a mismatch. This is an illustration of the matching hypothesis.

The two most common ways of investigating client-treatment interactions are the predictor approach and the differential approach. The former examines a single treatment (e.g., disulfiram) and examines individual differences to determine which ones might predict outcome. The differential approach compares two treatments within the same study and looks for differential predictors of success. The latter approach, while more difficult to do, results in

FIGURE 1. A hypothetical client-by-treatment interaction

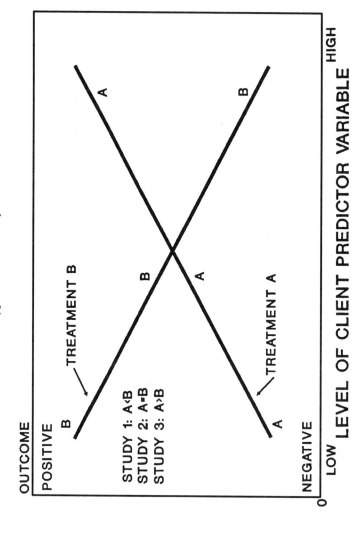

Reprinted with permission from W. R. Miller and N. Heather, (Eds.), *Treating Addictive Behaviors: Processes of Change*. New York: Plenum.

much more potentially useful clinical data about which types of clients respond best to which kinds of treatments.

Predictor studies have provided some initial and tantalizing information about how individual differences are related to specific treatments: psychotropic medications, disulfiram, Alcoholics Anonymous, psychotherapy, chemical aversion therapy, covert sensitization, relaxation training, social skills training, family therapy, the Community Reinforcement Approach, and Behavioral Self-Control Training. Differential studies have also started to document interactions with somewhat greater precision. The following matching variables have some data to suggest that they interact with treatment outcomes: problem severity, cognitive style, neuropsychological status, self-esteem, social stability, client choice, and other life problems. Miller & Hester (1986c) provide a review of the matching literature.

ASSESSING AND MOTIVATING PATIENTS TO BEGIN TREATMENT

Unless clients are motivated to do something about their drinking or drug use, a great deal of groundwork must be done before you attempt to match a client to a particular treatment. Rather than just starting off with an assessment or making a referral for treatment, it is important to judge where the person is in the process of change. Prochaska and DiClemente have developed an elegant model describing the processes of change. Initially based on case histories of individuals who quit smoking without formal treatment, this model has been validated as an accurate way to describe how people quit drinking and change other patterns of behavior (Prochaska and DiClemente, 1986). Figure 2 illustrates these stages and their relationship to each other.

Individuals in the Precontemplation Stage have not considered that their drinking or drug use may be presenting problems. When someone first discusses their drinking with them they might act surprised and puzzled.

More commonly, individuals with problems are in the Contemplation Stage. During this phase they are weighing the pros and

FIGURE 2. A stage model of the process of change; Prochaska and DiClemente.

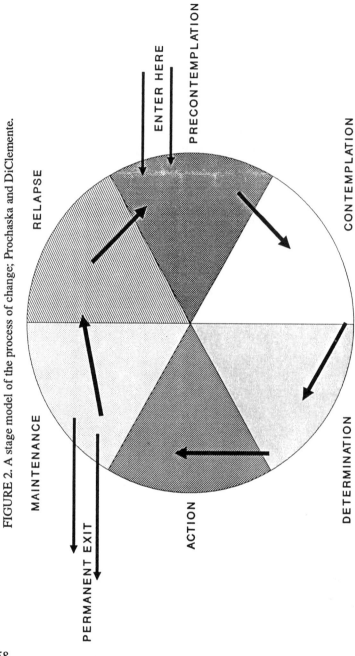

Reprinted with permission from Miller, W. R. and Jackson, K. A. (1985), *Practical Psychology for Counselors*, Englewood Cliffs, NJ: Prentice-Hall

cons of changing their behaviors. While they may acknowledge that their drinking has caused some problems, like a driving while intoxicated charge, for instance, they also say things like "but I don't drink in the morning," or "but, I don't drink any more than my friends do." A useful visual image of this phase is that of a seesaw. On one side a person puts all the good things he or she likes about drinking and what they might perceive are the bad things about not drinking. On the other side of the seesaw are all the problems drinking is causing and perceived positive benefits from not drinking. When the balance starts to consistently tip in favor of the negative consequences of drinking, a person moves toward determination to change. This is a process of attitudinal change in people.

The Determination Stage is thought of as a window of opportunity. If a person makes the decision to change, he or she will review the options available to see if they appear reasonable, are within his or her capabilities, and fit with his or her needs. People who find such an approach are likely to enter into and comply with the treatment.

The Action Stage is what most people think of as change. It is the period of time of actual drinking or drug behavior change. The Maintenance Stage is often the most difficult time, at least initially and requires different skills than those used to stop the drinking and drug use. As Mark Twain once said "Quitting smoking is easy. I've done it a thousand times."

The Relapse Stage is quite common. How a relapse or slip is dealt with by the individual, and his or her therapist if involved in aftercare, can have a strong influence on whether an individual returns to his or her previous patterns of heavy drinking or drug use. After a relapse, individuals often reassess their behaviors and situations and are again in the Contemplation Stage. They may then continue through the process of change again.

Matching issues are salient for individuals in the determination stage. If, as is more common, an individual is in the contemplation stage, you will need to figure out a way to help him or her move through that stage to determination. Until recently the most commonly accepted way to do this was to confront the person's denial and attempt to convince the person of the need to accept the label of "alcoholic" or "chemically dependent." Recent research, however, suggests that this approach may actually increase resistance to change (e.g., Miller & Sovereign, 1989). Instead, an alternative approach, now known as motivational interviewing (Miller, 1985) takes a much more indirect approach; yet recent data suggest that it is a more effective way to increase motivation for change (Miller & Sovereign, 1989).

MATCHING CLIENTS TO TREATMENTS: THE NEXT STEP

As a preface to this discussion, it is important to note that much of the current matching literature on client characteristics and specific interventions may be appropriate for individuals with physical and cognitive disabilities. Obviously, different patients will have different levels of problem severity, different cognitive styles and conceptual abilities, varying degrees of self-esteem, and different levels of social support.

In an attempt to clarify the following discussion, the assumption is made that patients who are being considered for referral to treatment for chemical dependency have been or still are in an acute rehabilitation center. If so, the question is usually not how to help patients stop drinking or using drugs because they have already been abstinent for perhaps several weeks to months. The question, then, is how to prevent relapse. A number of world class researchers (e.g., Helen Annis, Alan Marlatt) have developed theories of relapse prevention and specific interventions to address this phase of the process of change (Annis & Davis, 1989; Marlatt & Gordon, 1985).

In some instances clients who are being considered for referral for treatment are currently drinking and/or using drugs to varying degrees. This would be more common in outpatient rehabilitation centers. For these individuals, referrals to treatment approaches designed to halt the abuse are appropriate.

Currently no data have been published which provide clear guidelines about how best to match clients with physical and cognitive disabilities to various treatments. Indeed, this whole area is just beginning to evolve. Consequently the hypotheses about matching these populations must be considered speculative.

One way to conceptualize a patient's cognitive and physical disabilities is that of a life problem. Relevant questions include: How well is the individual coping with his or her disability, adapting to the changes, and returning to a productive, functional life? The extent to which a patient is adequately dealing with his or her disability influences the presence or absence of negative emotional states such as depression. Recent research in relapse prevention (Marlatt & Gordon, 1985) has found that the presence of negative emotional states is the single most common antecedent to relapse in heavy drinkers and alcoholics. Therefore training in appropriate disability coping skills (e.g., disability-specific assertiveness training) and strategies to manage and reduce depression (e.g., Beck's cognitive therapy) may substantially reduce the probability of relapse. This training is probably best done at the rehabilitation center unless a drug and alcohol abuse treatment center has specific expertise in these areas.

A second general consideration is that of social support for alcohol and drug abuse. If an individual is likely to return to a social network which encourages or condones alcohol and other drug abuse, the probability of relapse increases. If a patient is motivated to remain clean and sober, specific assertiveness training to resist these social pressures may prove helpful. Equipped with adequate skills and confidence, a patient will quickly find out which friends are supportive and which are simply drinking buddies who are threatened by or hostile to the patient's sobriety or reduced consumption. While initially it may be wise to avoid situations and places where patients used to drink heavily or use drugs, eventually and gradually they may need to learn the necessary skills to cope with those situations and settings without resorting to excessive drinking or drug use (see Annis and Davis, 1989, for a review of this approach and specific training strategies). If social pressures to drink heavily or use drugs are a concern, it is advisable to carefully investigate claims of treatment centers that they provide this kind of training. Referring parties should ask if they provide specific behavioral rehearsal, use a treatment manual or outline, and provide repeated opportunities to shape and train these skills. If possible, sitting in on a group involved in this training may be helpful to become acquainted with a treatment program's focus. If the training talks about assertiveness but does little, if any, behavioral rehearsal or training, it is unlikely to benefit your client. While some emphasis on cognitions which impede or prevent assertiveness is appropriate, a strictly insight-oriented approach is not as effective.

Interpersonal conflicts are another important antecedent to relapse. For some individuals drinking or drug use precipitates marital or family arguments. For others, however, the converse is true. If marital or family conflict continues in the absence of drinking or drug use, it should be addressed expeditiously. Behavioral marital therapy has been supported by controlled research as an effective intervention both for drinking and as a means to improve the marital relationship (O'Farrell & Cowes, 1989).

COGNITIVE DYSFUNCTIONS

The matching literature has documented an inverse relationship between levels of neuropsychological deficits and outcomes from treatment. Typically, however, the deficits have been a result of heavy drinking over a number of years. Thus these patients present a different picture than those of patients with head injuries and cerebral vascular accidents (CVAs). To date, no published studies have investigated matching clients to treatments who have had head injuries or CVAs.

Patients with brain injuries and those with CVAs generally constitute two distinct groups; young patients with head injuries and older adults who have CVAs. Patients with head injuries often have difficulty with attention and concentration skills, short-term memory and problem-solving abilities, communication and comprehension skills. These may be important factors in matching patients to the level of conceptual complexity of a program or intervention. The more concrete a patient's conceptual skills, the more contingency-based and concrete an intervention needs to be. Degree of emotional and impulse control also needs to be considered. Patients with significant problems with emotional or behavioral outbursts may not be well managed in traditional treatment programs. A behaviorally-oriented program which is knowledgeable about contingency management techniques would be better equipped for this task.

Patients with CVAs may also be at risk for developing problems with alcohol or drugs and may be particularly more prone to developing dependencies on prescription medications. This population appears to be at increased risk for clinical depression which may in turn increase their risk for abuse of alcohol and other drugs (Robinson & Price, 1982). Careful management by the patient's attending physician may prevent some problems with prescription medication abuse.

MAINTAINING CONTACT WITH REFERRED PATIENTS

It is important to realize, and to inform patients you refer to treatment, that the criteria for matching of clients to treatments are not perfect. Thus, the need to maintain contact with patients long after treatment has finished is apparent. If relapse occurs, it can signal that the patient may need some different type of intervention or training to deal with the events which precipitated the relapse in the first place. Unfortunately, too many treatment centers seem to be prone to provide similar treatments to patients when they might benefit from a variety of different treatments.

Following patients after treatment also allows you to develop a sense for which patients work best with which programs in your community. If your organization conducts follow-up research it could economically incorporate alcoholism treatment and outcome into its database and eventually enable you to develop decision trees for matching patients to treatments. This, in turn, holds great promise for improving the effectiveness and efficiency of treatment for your patients.

REFERENCES

Annis, H.M., & Davis, C.S. (1989). Relapse prevention. In R.K. Hester & W.R. Miller (Eds.), *Handbook of alcoholism treatment: Effective alternatives* (pp. 170- 182). Elmsford, NY: Pergamon.
McLachlan, J.F.C. (1974). Therapy strategies, personality orientation and recovery from alcoholism. *Canadian Psychiatric Association Journal, 19*, 25-30.

Marlatt, G.A., & Gordon, J.R. (1985). *Relapse Prevention*. NewYork: Guilford.

Miller, W.R. (1985). Motivation for treatment. A review with special emphasis on alcoholism. *Psychological Bulletin, 98*, 84-107.

Miller, W.R., & Hester, R.K. (1980). Treating the problem drinker: Modern approaches. In W.R. Miller (Ed.), *The addictive behaviors: Treatment of alcoholism, drug abuse, smoking, and obesity* (pp. 11-141). London: Pergamon.

Miller, W.R., & Hester, R.K. (1986a). The effectiveness of treatment techniques: What the research reveals. In W.R. Miller & N. Heather (Eds.), *Treating addictive behaviors: Processes of change* (pp. 121-174). New York: Plenum.

Miller, W.R. & Hester, R.K. (1986b). Inpatient alcoholism treatment: Who benefits? *American Psychologist, 41*, 794-805.

Miller, W.R., & Hester, R.K. (1986c). Matching problem drinkers with optimal treatments. In W.R. Miller & N. Heather (Eds.), *Treating addictive behaviors: Processes of change* (pp.175-204). New York: Plenum.

Miller, W.R., & Sovereign, R.G. (1989). The check-up: A model for early intervention in addictive behaviors. In T. Loberg, W.R. Miller, P.E. Nathan, & G.A. Marlatt (Eds.), *Addictive behaviors: Prevention and early intervention* (pp. 219-231). Amsterdam: Swets & Zeitlinger.

O'Farrell, T.J., & Cowes, K.S. (1989). Marital and family therapy. In R.K. Hester & W.R. Miller (Eds.), *Handbook of alcoholism treatment: Effective alternatives* (pp. 183-205). Elmsford, NY: Pergamon.

Prochaska, J.O., & DiClemente, C.C. (1986). Toward a comprehensive model of change. In W.R. Miller & N. Heather (Eds.), *Treating addictive behaviors: Processes of change* (pp. 3-27). New York: Plenum.

Robinson, R.G., & Price, T.R. (1982). Poststroke depressive disorders: A follow-up study of 103 patients. *Stroke, 13*, 635-641.

Chapter 12

Chemical Dependency: The Avoided Issue for Persons with Physical Disabilities

Sharon Schaschl, RN, BSN, CCDP
Dennis Straw, CCDP

For many persons with physical disabilities, chemical dependency imposes far greater limitations than does their physical impairment (O'Donnell et al., 1981-1982). Until recently, the need for chemical dependency treatment and the benefits of recovery for persons with disabilities have not been acknowledged by society, the medical community, families, and peer groups (Dufour et al., 1989). Failure to adequately address chemical dependency as a primary health care issue will prevent successful rehabilitation and disability adjustment, lead to increased medical complications of the disability, and interfere with independent living.

Often the problems caused by chemical dependency are attributed to the disability and a great deal of time, energy, and money may be spent treating symptoms rather than the disease of chemical dependency. These misdirected efforts will result in little positive change for the person with a physical disability and considerable stress for concerned persons who may experience feelings of frustration, inadequacy, and anger, as well as physical and emotional exhaustion. Persons who are aware of the relationship between chemical dependency and disability and are willing to address chemical use issues, are able to facilitate a change to a productive lifestyle for persons with disabilities who are experiencing problems as a result of their chemical use.

CHEMICAL DEPENDENCY AS A PRIMARY HEALTH CARE ISSUE

Chemical dependency is recognized by the American Medical Association as a chronic, progressive disease. The disease may be manifested by the onset of problems in any or all areas of a person's life and will ultimately lead to death if left untreated. Although there is no cure for this disease and it will not spontaneously resolve, recovery is possible, but involves more than merely limiting chemical use. Recovery is achieved through abstinence from mood-altering chemicals, participation in a treatment program, and ongoing support. The disease cannot be treated by attempts to resolve other identified problems which may be attributed to the disability. Those problems are usually the result of the chemical dependency and cannot be resolved until the chemical dependency is treated.

FACTORS WHICH PERPETUATE CHEMICAL DEPENDENCY

Major factors which perpetuate the high rate of chemical dependency for persons with disabilities include the negative attitudes commonly held toward both disability and chemical dependency, myths regarding the cause and effect relationship of disability and chemical dependency, enabling of persons with disabilities by the medical community, family, and friends, lack of knowledge and skills regarding the relationship between chemical dependency and physical disability, and the lack of specialized treatment programs.

Attitudes

The most significant of these factors appears to be the negative attitudes commonly held toward both disability and chemical dependency. Persons with disabilities are often considered hopeless, helpless, fragile, pitiful, and sick (Hepner, Kirshbaum, & Landes, 1980-1981). Disability is commonly equated with illness, thus fostering the idea that persons with disabilities are incapable of assuming responsibility for themselves, require repeated hospitalizations, and must depend on some type of mood-altering medication in order to function. Family, friends, and the medical community often feel that there is little value for persons with disabilities in achieving a chemically-free lifestyle, as the chemicals are seen as a justifiable means of masking reality. It is assumed that without these chemicals persons with disabilities could not cope with what is perceived as a miserable existence.

Furthermore, family, friends and the medical community are reluctant to associate the shameful implications of chemical dependency with the victim of a disability. Dealing with chemical dependency is seen as an extra burden, and chemical dependency treatment for persons with disabilities is frequently viewed as cruel, unfair, and a waste of time and money.

Myths

One common myth which may perpetuate chemical dependency is the belief that disability causes chemical dependency. People do not become chemically dependent because of a crisis, although a crisis may prompt increased chemical use. For persons who have congenital disabilities and are chemically dependent, the chemical dependency was not created by the disability. Many received mood-altering medications since childhood and were living in protective environments which controlled their chemical use. Persons with congenital disabilities with whom we have worked have indicated that when they left these environments and attempted to integrate into an able-bodied society, increased chemical use became an equalizer and chemical dependency flourished. For persons whose disabilities were the result of a later-onset trauma or illness, research clearly indicates that the majority were having problems related to their use of mood-altering chemicals long before the onset of their disability (United States Department of Education, 1982; O'Donnell et al., 1981-1982). Statistics from the Chemical Dependency/Physical Disability Program at Abbott Northwestern Hospital/Sister Kenny Institute indicate that of the patients admitted for chemical dependency treatment approximately 80% with later-onset disabilities were chemically dependent prior to the onset of their disabilities; the use of mood-altering chemicals was a contributing factor to accident or illness for approximately the same proportion (Schaschl & Straw, 1989).

A second myth is the belief that disability is the primary cause of problems for persons with disabilities. Persons who abuse chemicals will function well below their potential and will experience problems in many areas of their lives: physical, emotional, spiritual, social, family, and other relationships, sexual, legal, vocational, and financial. These problems may be manifested by frequent health problems and hospitalizations, low self-esteem, poor personal hygiene, dependent lifestyle, association primarily with chemical users, lack of motivation, significant personality changes, memory deficits, depression, suicide attempts, departure from personal values, rejection of beliefs that once were important, isolation from family and friends, involvement in unhealthy relationships, sexual abuse, inappropriate sexual behavior, poor body image, arrests, incarceration, loss of driver's license or public transportation privileges, drug-dealing, unemployment, failure in school, lack of vocational involvement, and difficulty meeting basic financial obligations. Problems such as these are usually attributed to the disability as concerned persons may not recognize the possibility that chemical use is a significant contributing factor.

Enabling

Enabling chemical use by the medical community, family, and friends occurs in an effort to protect persons with disabilities from the reality of their disability. In other words, chemical use may be seen as a way to ease the pain and take their minds off their troubles. Enabling of chemical use also serves to alleviate the enabler's own uncomfortable feelings about the disability. As the person with a physical disability appears to escape an unpleasant reality under the influence of mood-altering chemicals, enablers can believe they are helping, and all can avoid dealing with the disability on an honest, emotional level.

A physical disability may legitimize the prescription of mood-altering medications, but as the symptoms of the disability (e.g., pain and spasticity) persist, these acute medications may be inappropriately prescribed on a long-term basis by physicians who may feel helpless and frustrated because they cannot fix the disability (United States Department of Education, 1990). Often it becomes apparent that medications which have been prescribed for pain or spasticity may also relieve disability-related feelings of fear, anger, rejection, inadequacy, frustration or sadness. The continued use of these mood- altering medications is welcomed. Alcohol use may be condoned, and may even be prescribed within medical facilities, despite the known depressive effects of alcohol, a history of chemical abuse, and possible adverse interaction with medications.

It is commonly assumed that persons with disabilities who are chemically dependent are primarily addicted to medications which were prescribed because of the disability. For the majority of patients in the Chemical Dependency/Physical Disability Program at Abbott Northwestern Hospital/Sister Kenny Institute in Minneapolis, the drug of choice has been alcohol, usually in combination with marijuana or other street drugs (Schaschl & Straw, 1989). Prescription medications, which are easily obtained and are usually paid for by third party reimbursement, are frequently used as a substitute or alternative when the drug of choice is not available; medications may be sold or exchanged for the drug of choice. For chemically dependent persons, disability can be a ticket to manipulate the medical community into prescribing not only mood-altering medications, but specifically those which are preferred.

Finally, friends and the medical community may change their values regarding chemical use when a person with a physical disability is involved. Behaviors which are unacceptable for a nondisabled person may be permitted, ignored, or excused for someone who has a disability. Chemical use may be viewed and encouraged as a means of socializing and achieving equality with able-bodied friends, as "one of the few sources of pleasure" for a person with a physical disability, and as an escape from the reality of the disability (Brubeck, 1981). Enablers may profess that they have no right to deny persons with disabilities their choices, even if those choices are self-destructive. However, enablers often lose sight of their own choices as they provide the person with a physical disability with permission or assistance needed to carry out the destructive behavior.

Relationship Between Chemical Dependency and Physical Disability

The lack of knowledge and skills regarding the relationship between chemical dependency and physical disability allows considerable time, energy, and money to be spent addressing disability-related issues while the person with a physical disability makes little progress toward a more productive and satisfying lifestyle. Any use of mood-altering chemicals by persons with disabilities will medicate the feelings related to their disability. These feelings are a natural part of the grieving process and must be experienced in order to accept disability as nondevaluing. Persons with disabilities may appear to express their feelings, but the chemicals will prevent integration of logical thoughts and emotions into a unified acceptance of the disability.

Addressing Chemical Use Issues with Persons with Disabilities

Persons with disabilities must have access to chemical use information, early chemical dependency evaluation, intervention and appropriate treatment. It is essential that persons with disabilities receive chemical use education as a regular component of their rehabilitation program. This information is equally important to the person with a disability, family, friends, and caregivers. Ideally, providing this information simultaneously to all persons involved may prevent misunderstandings about the use of mood-altering chemicals, limit enabling, and begin to establish a support system. Persons with disabilities need specific information about the effects of chemicals as they relate to the disability, the interaction of medications, alcohol and other drugs, the disease of chemical dependency and its warning signs, and resources for accessing help. When a chemical use problem is indicated or suspected, it is essential to arrange for a chemical use evaluation with the expectation that the recommendations will be followed (National Institute on Alcohol Abuse and Alcoholism, 1989).

In working with providers of chemical dependency services, it is essential to utilize professionals who are knowledgeable and skilled in working with persons with disabilities. Documentation from rehabilitation professionals relating to chemical use can be valuable to the evaluator; collateral contact with concerned persons who have information about the individual's chemical use is essential. If the evaluation indicates the need for chemical dependency treatment, this may begin as soon as the individual is medically stable. Usually treatment is postponed until the acute rehabilitation phase is completed unless the chemical use is interfering with that process. Frequently it is assumed that a person should have emotionally adjusted to his or her disability before entering treatment. Unfortunately, disability adjustment is one of the primary areas which is stalled by chemical use; addressing the chemical use may be the only way to facilitate the disability adjustment process.

Persons with physical disabilities who are referred for chemical dependency treatment need not only architectural accessibility, but ideally a specific physical disability program coordinated by professionals experienced in both chemical dependency and physical disability, and knowledgeable about community resources.

Issues to be considered in evaluating and treating persons with disabilities for chemical dependency include: the attitudes commonly held toward disability by patient, staff, and family; architectural accessibility; financial accessibility; the need for assistance with personal care; level of disability adjustment; use of medications; management of chronic pain, spasticity, and stress; communication; ability to perform required program activities; access to adaptive exercise, recreation, and relaxation; support systems; self-pity and learned helplessness (Davidson, 1983); manipulative skill (Anderson, 1980-1981); lack of history of meaningful activity; and aftercare resources. While these issues may warrant program adaptations in order to assure full participation, they do not justify special privileges which will create resentment among other patients.

Persons with disabilities who have difficulties with reading, writing, communication, or who have limited ability to perform the tasks required by the program are entitled to adaptations such as reading materials on audio tapes; a tape recorder for dictating written assignments; staff members available for written dictation; assistance with laundry, cleaning or other activities; and adaptive recreation, exercise, and relaxation.

Often persons with disabilities have not been expected to assume responsibility for themselves or their actions, and have learned to respond to the low expectations of others with self-pity, learned helplessness, or manipulation. Most chemically dependent persons with disabilities have no history of productive activity since the onset of their disabilities, and they see little hope for a meaningful lifestyle in the future without the use of mood-altering chemicals. Failure to acknowledge abilities allows persons with disabilities to avoid active and equal participation in the treatment process.

Many chemically dependent persons with disabilities do not have healthy support systems. They may have burned out their families, may be living with attendants who are using or enabling, and may associate primarily with other people who are using. Without a supportive living environment outpatient treatment, aftercare and sustained recovery are very difficult. Finding a safe place to live after treatment may be impossible. Long waiting lists confront patients who wish to relocate to accessible housing; inaccessibility may prohibit a temporary stay with a sober friend while relocating; and few halfway houses are accessible.

Medications are viewed in two different categories: convenience and essential. Addictive, mood-altering muscle relaxants to control spasticity and narcotics to manage chronic pain are viewed as convenience medications. Anticonvulsants to control seizures are viewed as essential medications. Mood-altering, addictive medications are inappropriate when used to treat chronic conditions. Antidepressants are appropriate when used in conjunction with counseling and medical supervision. Chemically dependent persons with disabilities need to develop alternate methods of managing chronic pain, spasticity and stress. Relaxation, meditation, acupressure, biofeedback, self-hypnosis, diet, exercise, stretching, hot packs, cold packs, whirlpool, and massage are effective replacement techniques. The techniques may be developed independently or as part of a formal chronic pain rehabilitation program. For persons who become chemically free, there seems to be approximately a three-month period following withdrawal of chemicals during which pain and spasticity seem intensified as adequate endorphin levels have not yet been reestablished and the nervous system is adjusting to its unmedicated state. A great deal of emotional support is needed at this time as this is commonly the period during which patients return to their physicians requesting and receiving medications.

For chemically dependent persons with disabilities, the chemical use has allowed them to remain in a state of denial, anger or depression about their disabilities. The use of mood-altering chemicals prevents persons with disabilities from experiencing feelings related to their disabilities. Those feelings are a natural part of the grieving process and must be experienced if the person is to integrate thoughts and emotions in a unified process of disability adjustment.

Without consideration of these issues, chemical dependency treatment for persons with disabilities may not be maximally effective and the opportunity for successful recovery may be limited.

THE PROFESSIONAL'S ROLE

Professionals who understand the significance of chemical dependency as a primary health care issue and are aware of the indicators of chemical dependency for persons with disabilities are in a position to intervene on a chemical use problem. Professionals must become aware of their own attitudes towards chemical dependency and persons with disabilities. They must examine their own as well as their family's and friends' patterns of chemical use. If they, or someone close to them, abuse chemicals, it will be difficult to see or confront the patient's chemical use. Someone who views chemical dependency as a moral weakness or a self-inflicted condition may not work as effectively with an addict as someone who has a healthy understanding of the disease of chemical dependency. Negative attitudes will be apparent to patients, will raise their psychological defenses, and will increase their emotional distance. Changing attitudes is difficult; but self-reflection in conjunction with education about chemical dependency and its effects on a person's life may facilitate the process. A support network is important for anyone who chooses to address the issue of chemical dependency. This network is essential in validating concerns, formulating plans and dealing with patients' responses. Often a chemically dependent person may instigate conflict between team members to prevent recognition of a chemical use problem.

Professionals who have done this background work are now in a position to address chemical dependency issues with patients. The first step is observation. Professionals must become aware of what is heard, seen, and smelled; they must trust their instincts. Sometimes it may be nothing more than a gut feeling that something is not quite right. It is essential that observations be documented. If patients are heard talking about the consequences of their drug use, it should be documented. If deterioration in performance or attitude is observed, it should be documented. If the smell of alcohol is apparent on someone's breath, it should be documented. Documentation should be objective descriptions of observations, not judgments, analyses or conclusions. An appropriate example may be: "I smelled alcohol on John's breath this morning. His eyes appeared glassy and his speech was slurred." Observations should be shared with the patient, and the patient's response should be documented: "I told John I smelled alcohol on his breath and he said it was his new mouthwash." If the patient does not have a problem, this may be the only incident ever documented. If the patient does have a chemical use problem, a pattern will emerge. It is most beneficial to both patients and staff to have programs and institutions develop chemical use policies with a therapeutic option for chemical dependency evaluation and treatment. Given the increased risk of chemical abuse for persons with disabilities, it is useful to conduct basic screening for chemical abuse with every patient.

A MODEL PROGRAM

In 1983, Abbott Northwestern Hospital/Sister Kenny Institute in Minneapolis implemented an innovative Chemical Dependency/ Physical Disability Program designed to meet the special needs of persons with disabilities. The program staff includes a Program Coordinator who is a Certified Chemical Dependency Practitioner and an experienced rehabilitation nurse, and a Program Consultant who is a Certified Chemical Dependency Practitioner, has a physical disability, and is recovering from chemical dependency. The program staff is an integral part of the treatment team; their work focuses on three distinct areas. On the physical rehabilitation units at Sister Kenny Institute and in the Chronic Pain Rehabilitation Program, the program staff provides chemical dependency evaluations, consultation and education to patients, staff and families.

On the physical rehabilitation units and in the Chronic Pain Rehabilitation Program at Sister Kenny Institute, the program staff provides chemical dependency evaluations for patients. Through a series of lectures, group discussions, and interactive exercises, the program staff provides patients and families with attitude awareness and information on medications and other chemicals. They provide support and consultation for families. They offer consultation and education to staff to enable them to deal effectively with chemical use and to develop and implement chemical use policies. They also offer assistance with interventions.

In the community, the program staff conducts workshops throughout the country to increase awareness of the issue of chemical abuse for persons with disabilities, and provide direction in identifying, addressing and referring chemically dependent persons with physical disabilities. They are also involved in consultation for program development.

The counseling and nursing staff in the chemical dependency treatment center have a working knowledge of the interrelationship between chemical dependency and physical disability. They also coordinate a disability component which has been integrated into Abbott Northwestern Hospital's Chemical Dependency Treatment Program. The rationale for establishing the disability component was based on the premise that a disability is a significant fact which needs to be addressed in order to facilitate recovery. The person's disability has been a primary factor to justify chemical use, and unresolved issues surrounding the disability will continue to be a ticket to continue or resume chemical use. The Program Coordinator and Program Consultant provide evaluation, intervention and referral services, assistance with program adaptations, individual counseling and support to patients and their families for disability and dependency issues, and, with two other professionals, facilitate a weekly peer-support group for recovering persons with disabilities. The program staff offers counselors and medical staff assistance in addressing the disability as it relates to treating the primary illness of chemical dependency. Program staff facilitates communication with referral sources at patient's or counselor's request to formulate and implement aftercare plans which incorporate disability and dependency issues. Additionally, the program staff offers follow-up consultations, education, and awareness training as necessary to reintegrate the person with a physical disability into the community.

Patients with disabilities usually comprise five to ten percent of the total patient population. They are expected to participate with nondisabled patients in all program activities as scheduled. Adaptations are made to accommodate physical limitations in order to assure full participation. For patients who require personal care service, a home health care agency schedules certified nursing assistants for two-hour periods in the morning and evening. Nursing care, treatments, medications and any additional assistance throughout the day are provided by the regular nursing staff. Physical therapy and occupational therapy are ordered only if necessary to maintain the patient's level of function.

An important element of the program is the weekly Chemical Dependency/Physical Disability Support Group which is facilitated by four professionals who are experienced in both chemical dependency and physical disability. The group first met in August, 1983, with one member and three facilitators. Attendance has steadily increased and has maintained a consistent weekly attendance of 18 to 25 participants over the past two years. At present, there are 20 active core members. Length of membership ranges from two weeks to four years; sobriety ranges from two weeks to 14 years. The age range of members is 20 to 53 years, with the average being approximately 34 years.

The group is available for persons with disabilities for whom the use of alcohol or drugs has been a problem and who wish to pursue a more meaningful lifestyle without the use of mood-altering chemicals. The group's rules are simple: members must have a disability and a desire to remain free of all mood-altering chemicals. Although it is expected that group members will attend a 12-step group on a regular basis in addition to this group, some members find it difficult to do this initially, and need time to put their disabilities into perspective.

Many patients with disabilities have been resistant to participating in the group, and most were required to attend initially. Strong denial has been evident when patients with severe disabilities refused to attend the group stating, "I've already adjusted to my disability," "I'm not like those people," "It depresses me to be around those people," and "What right do you have to label me 'disabled'?" For patients who readily attended the group for the first time, it was frequently with the expectation that they would receive support for their chemical use from those who understood its justification. These patients were disappointed and frustrated when the group's support and understanding were focused on their feelings relating to their disability and the merits of achieving a chemically-free lifestyle. Group members provide role models on how to live with a physical disability without medicating every physical and emotional symptom. Participation becomes voluntary when there is a willingness to address the disability and identify with the group.

The group generates discussion about disability issues which were not appropriate to discuss in regular treatment groups or other 12-step meetings. Each member is encouraged to deal with his or her own issues, and is allowed to do so in his or her own time. The peer support from a diverse group of people and their experiences is what provides fertile grounds for personal growth. The group provides support and stimulates creative thinking as members begin integrating into a nondisabled society. Each new achievement by an individual geometrically increases the data base of the whole group.

For many group members, the group has become an important part of their recoveries as evidenced in their commitment to attend. Several members have had multiple treatments and are finally maintaining an extended period of sobriety. For the first time they are addressing their disabilities, an element which was missing from previous treatment experiences.

OUTCOMES

Those persons who have chosen to remain chemically free and to become actively involved in a recovery program gain self-esteem, self-respect, and self-responsibility, and begin the process of accepting their disabilities. They experience better health, and develop alternative means of managing chronic pain, sleep disorders, spasticity and stress. New social experiences replace isolation, and healthy relationships replace abusive, dependent ones. Many have developed more independent lifestyles, become involved in vocational and avocational activities, and resolve financial and legal difficulties. This pattern has been observed in other settings as well (Sweeney & Foote, 1982).

There appears to be a direct correlation between remaining actively connected to the Disability Support Group and prolonged, meaningful recovery. Of 112 patients admitted to our program from June 1, 1983, to February 29, 1988, 29 were known to be recovering, and 25 of these 29 persons attended group on a regular basis for at least 12 weeks. Five out-of-state patients attended four times regularly while in treatment. The range of sobriety was from nine months to five years. Most of our patients have coped with their disabilities through the use of chemicals, and regardless of duration of disability, the grieving process had been arrested. Persons who resumed their chemical use have not been able to engage in the process of adjusting to disability and those who have not engaged in the process of adjusting to their disability have resumed their chemical use. Forty of the 112 patients were known to have relapsed. Persons who have been willing to address both their dependency and their disability, and work through the acceptance process with each, have had the greatest success in recovery.

The first eight years of the program have proved a formidable challenge and a tremendous learning experience. The valuable knowledge and expertise we have gained have enabled us to provide assistance in program development, educational workshops addressing the issue of chemical dependency and disability, and a resource for chemical dependency evaluation and treatment for persons with disabilities. We are grateful to our patients who have allowed us to be a part of their recovery process.

REFERENCES

Anderson, P. (Winter 1980-1981). Alcoholism and the spinal cord disabled: A model program. *Alcohol Health and Research World*, 37-41.

Brubeck, T. (November-December 1981). Alcoholism–The extra burden. *American Rehabilitation*, 7(2), 3-6.

Davidson, W. (Fall, 1983). Babying the handicapped. *IPT Newsletter*, 6-7.

Dufour, M., et al. (1989). Alcohol-related morbidity among the disabled. *Alcohol, Health and Research World, 13*(2), 158-161.

Hepner, R., Kirshbaum, H., & Landes, D. (Winter, 1980-1981). Counseling substance abusers with additional disabilities: The center for independent living. *Alcohol Health and Research World, 5*(2), 11-13.

National Institute on Alcohol Abuse and Alcoholism, United States Department of Health and Human Services (1989). Alcohol and trauma. *Alcohol Alert*, Number 3.

O'Donnell, J., et al. (Winter, 1981-1982). Alcohol, drugs and spinal cord injury. *Alcohol Health and Research World, 6*(2), 27-20.

Schaschl, S., & Straw, D. (1989). Results of a model intervention program for physically impaired persons. *Alcohol Health and Research World*, United States Department of Health and Human Services Publication No. (ADM), *13*(2), 89-153.

Sweeney, T., & Foote, J. (1982). Treatment of drug and alcohol abuse in spinal cord injury veterans. *The International Journal of Addictions, 17*(5), 897-904.

United States Department of Education, Office of Special Education and Rehabilitation services (1982). Alcoholism as a secondary disability: The silent saboteur in rehabilitation. *Rehab Brief, 5*(6).

United States Department of Education, Office of Special Education and Rehabilitation Services (1990). Substance abuse and disability. *Rehab Brief, 12*(12).

Chapter 13

Institute on Alcohol, Drugs, and Disability: From Grassroots Activity to Systems Changes

Linda Cherry, BA

This chapter is offered as an example of how concerned individuals working together can create changes in political and service systems. It chronicles a grassroots effort in the San Francisco Bay Area that used public and private resources, survey research and coalition building to create greater accessibility to alcohol and other drug treatment and recovery programs. Leadership continues in identifying and remediating all alcohol and other drug problems affecting people with disabilities.

The Institute on Alcohol, Drugs and Disability (IADD, formerly the Coalition on Disability and Chemical Dependency–CDCD) is a voluntary group of Bay Area service providers and consumers. The organization began in 1984 when 30 professionals from the alcohol and drug and the disability service fields met at Stanford University to plan a major conference on disability and chemical dependency. That conference convened in November, 1984 at the California School for the Deaf in Fremont. The consensus of the 100 participants supported the organizing premise of the conference that problems with alcohol and other drugs were a major, unaddressed issue among people with disabilities. In addition, it was agreed that major deficits existed in appropriate information and technical support for both individuals and potential service providers. That conference also developed the Disabilities/Substance Abuse Task Force which met regularly over the next two years. The work of the task force was carried out through donations of time and funds from its members and contributions from disability service agencies and alcohol and drug programs.

In mid-1986, the Disabilities/Substance Abuse Task Force incorporated into the nonprofit Coalition on Disability and Chemical Dependency. CDCD's Board of Directors included professionals from disability services at post-secondary educational institutions, independent living centers, the California Department of Rehabilitation, alcohol and drug programs, consumer groups and regional developmental disabilities centers as well as a lawyer, psychologist and architectural accessibility consultant. CDCD changed its name to the Institute on Alcohol, Drugs and Disability in 1989 to reflect its expanded vision and goals.

During its first years, IADD represented the issue of alcohol and other drug problems among people with disabilities through information booths at the Alameda County Department of Alcohol and Drug Program's Staying Alive '86 health fair and at the New Visions Resources for the Disabled community fair in San Mateo County. A newsletter, *The Seed,* was established as a forum on issues of access to alcohol and other drug treatment and recovery services for individuals with disabilities.

IADD sponsored a second conference in June, 1986. This conference, Confronting the Issues, drew some 100 people. Sessions were designed to present disability issues to alcohol and drug service providers and, conversely, to present alcohol and other drug issues to providers of disability services. In other outreach and awareness activities, IADD board members conducted the workshop, Disability and Chemical Dependency, at the 1987 Forum on Chemical Dependency in Sacramento, and, under contract with the San Mateo County Alcohol and Drug Program, developed and implemented a specialized training workshop for community-based alcohol and drug service providers. This Ramps Are Not Enough! workshop was a unique effort to enlist alcohol and drug professionals in a collaborative effort with disability service agencies to improve linkages.

STAFFING REQUIRED

Although IADD had succeeded in creating an awareness of the issue of alcohol and other drug problems among people with disabilities, its voluntary board of directors felt that significant progress required an ongoing project with staff dedicated to furthering the goals of the organization. Toward that end, funding was sought and received from the San Francisco Foundation, the Atkinson Foundation and the County of San Mateo Department of Community Services to conduct the Bay Area Project on Disabilities and Chemical Dependency with the cosponsorship of the Center for Independence of the Disabled (CID) in Belmont.

CDCD engaged Social Marketing and Communications Consultant Linda Cherry to direct the Bay Area Project. Designed to improve access to treatment and recovery services, the Project had two principal goals:

1. To document the incidence and prevalence of alcohol and drug (both illicit and prescription) problems among adults with mobility, visual or hearing impairments in San Mateo, Alameda and Marin counties.
2. To provide advocacy and technical assistance to enable alcohol and drug programs and disability programs in those counties to improve their services with regard to this issue.

BAY AREA PROJECT ON DISABILITIES AND CHEMICAL DEPENDENCY

One of the objectives of the first phase of the Bay Area Project on Disabilities and Chemical Dependency was to survey agencies that provide alcohol and drug services or disability services about their experiences with and understanding of clients who have mobility, visual or hearing impairments as well as problems with alcohol or other drugs, either illicit or prescription.

Most alcohol and drug service providers surveyed were publicly funded. That is, a large part of their operating budgets are provided through contracts with county or state agencies. In addition, programs that were under contract with each county to conduct drinking driver programs were also surveyed. The decision to focus on publicly-funded programs had several rationales. One was economic. Many people with disabilities, and especially those who also have alcohol or drug problems, may not have the financial resources for private treatment. Many private treatment programs are hospital-based, and there is a strong feeling within the disability community that people with physical (as well as mental or developmental) impairments have been *medicalized* enough. A community-based program that focuses on lifestyle, rather than clinical, issues seemed preferable.

In California, most publicly-funded alcohol and drug programs subscribe to many, if not all, of the concepts of such a social model philosophy. What is more, these publicly funded programs already operate under mandates to provide services to people with disabilities. Section 504 of the Rehabilitation Act of 1973 (Public Law Number 93-112), prohibits discrimination by any agency that receives federal assistance in providing services to people with disabilities. Virtually all programs with a county or state contract receive federal funding. The question, then, becomes: to what extent is the 504 mandate being followed?

A four-page, 74-item survey was developed by the Bay Area Project Director in consultation with three members from the Institute on Alcohol, Drugs and Disability Board of Directors (Bouquin, Zirpolo, and de Miranda; see IADD board list, Figure 1) who served as the Project Steering Committee. Input was also obtained from staff members of an alcohol program and the cosponsoring independent living center as well as from Project funding sources.

Introductory letters launching the Bay Area Project were distributed in January, 1988. Surveys, along with cover letters cosigned by the alcohol and drug program administrator in each county, were sent during the last week of February to service agencies and drinking driver programs operated by 35 corporations in the three counties. Reminder phone calls were made, and letters and duplicate surveys were sent to nonrespondents three weeks later. By the end of April, 30 programs representing 21 corporations returned completed surveys, a response rate of 60%.

Of the 30 respondents, some indicated more than one option within many of the data items. Others did not respond to certain items. Therefore, the percentages indicated in this report rarely total 100% for any one item. The percentages reflect the proportion of responses per item in relation to the entire 30 respondents.

FIGURE 1. IADD Board of Directors

James R. Bouquin
Disability Resource Center
123 Meyer Library
Stanford University
Stanford, CA 94305-3093
(415) 723-1039

Shirley Negrin
Department of Rehabilitation
2080 Tasso Street
Palo Alto, CA 94618
(415) 571-1311

A. Robert Balow, treasurer
Waddell & Reed Financial
    Services
3375 Scott Blvd., Suite 336
Santa Clara, CA 95054
(408) 496-6344

Christine Saulnier
6059 Johnston Drive
Berkeley, CA 94709
(415) 464-3430

Anthony Tusler, president
Disability Resource Center
Sonoma State University
Rohnert Park, CA 94928
(707) 664-2850

Christine Hoffman
Laney College Access Center
900 Fallon Street
Oakland, CA 94607
(415) 464-3428

Victor Colman, J.D.
Attorney
Santa Clara County Bureau
    of Alcohol Services
976 Lenzen Avenue
San Jose, CA 95126
(408) 299-6141

Jean Gillespie, secretary
Adult Independence
    Development Center
1190 Benton Street
Santa Clara, CA 95050
(408) 985-1243

Laura A. Soman
Health Care Consultant
3027 Wheeler Street
Berkeley, CA 94705
(415) 848-8859

IADD Consultants

Linda Cherry
3224 Round Hill Drive
Hayward, CA 04542
(415) 582-6838

John de Miranda
2165 Bunker Hill Drive
San Mateo, CA 94402
(415) 578-8047

Of initial interest was the attention given to the notion of providing services to people with disabilities. One way to determine an agency's interest in an issue is whether it provides staff training about that issue. Figure 2 shows that during the past year, staff training was offered in several areas by the alcohol and drug programs that responded to the survey. Programs offered by at least half of the agencies included working with people with AIDS, with families, ethnic minorities, pregnant women and youth. These findings suggest that little attention had been paid to people with disabilities and even less to older adults, another population likely to experience disabilities.

Service Statistics

Survey questions were also asked about the number of people with disabilities who contacted and were served by alcohol and drug programs during the most recent reporting year. Respondents indicated serving 21,122 individual adults on-site. They reported knowing of 246 individuals with disabilities who contacted them for services. Fifty-three percent of respondents indicated they do not keep records that allow them to determine the number of individuals with disabilities who were served. Services were provided to people with known disabilities in the following numbers:

- Mobility impairments   100 individuals
                             (0.47% of total client load)
- Mental disabilities   100 individuals (0.47%)
- Hearing impairments   59 individuals (0.28%)
- Developmental disabilities   39 individuals (0.18%)
- Visual impairments   36 individuals (0.17%)

In total, 334 individuals, or less than 1.6% of the total client population seen by respondents, were people with disabilities. Total population for the three counties surveyed is 2,097,563. The Department of Rehabilitation estimates that in any given population, 15% will have a disability. These percentages suggest that 314,634 individuals in Alameda, Marin, and San Mateo counties have disabilities. Traditional alcohol field estimates indicate that 10% of a

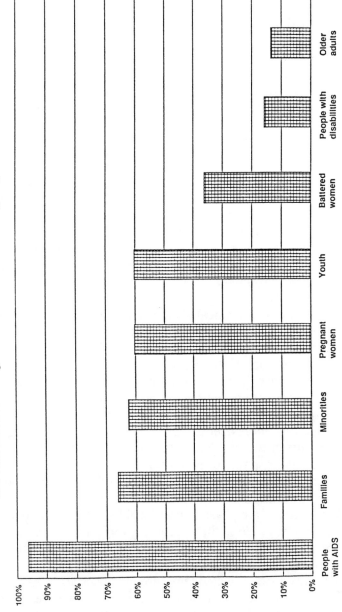

FIGURE 2. Staff Trainings Provided in Alcohol and Drug Programs in Past Year

The relative importance of issues can sometimes be evaluated by the attention those issues receive in an agency. This graph depicts the percentages of alcohol and drug programs that provided staff training on working with signifi-cant client populations during the past year.

population will have serious drinking problems, and another 10% can be expected to have problems with other drugs (illicit, prescription, over-the-counter, steroids, etc.). Considered together, these statistics suggest that 62,927 individuals with disabilities in Alameda, Marin, and San Mateo counties may also have problems with alcohol or other drugs. The 334 service recipients during the most recent reporting year, represent only 0.53% of those likely to be in need of services.

Barriers to Services

Figure 3 shows that respondents found the following major obstacles to their programs serving clients with disabilities: budget restraints, inaccessible facilities, program policy on medications, no client contacts for services, extra work requirements on staff, inconsistent licensing requirements, clients' failure to follow through, and a belief that disability diverts attention away from program goals and objectives.

Examination of the physical characteristics of respondents' facilities revealed that about half of them were totally or mostly accessible for those with mobility impairments. Figure 4 shows that accessibility was limited by 32-inch wide doorways, inadequate hallways, inadequate space in waiting rooms, inaccessible restrooms, appropriate ramps, entryways and parking.

While no question was asked about accessibility and usability of sleeping quarters in residential programs, many such programs often have quite crowded sleeping facilities and may be reluctant to relinquish the floor space necessary for a person using a wheelchair to maneuver so as to serve the most clients possible. The responses do suggest, however, that nearly half of alcohol and drug programs in the three counties are physically accessible to those with mobility impairments. The question then becomes: why so little service?

Sixty-seven percent of alcohol and drug respondents indicated they are totally or mostly accessible to those with visual impairments, but only 10% indicated they provide materials in large print or braille or that hazardous areas are marked. Thirty-seven percent indicated they are totally or mostly accessible for those with hearing impairments, but only 13% made sign language interpreters avail-

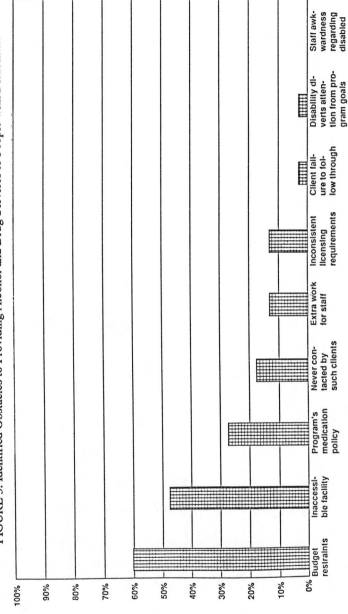

FIGURE 3. Identified Obstacles to Providing Alcohol and Drug Services to People with Disabilities

Alcohol and drug programs report a variety of major obstacles to their serving clients with disabilities. This graph shows the reported prevalence of such obstacles.

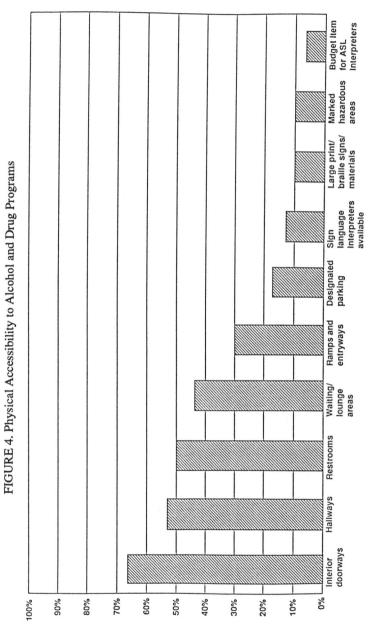

FIGURE 4. Physical Accessibility to Alcohol and Drug Programs

Physical accessibility to an alcohol or drug program requires more than a ramp to the entryway. This graph indicates the percentages of programs that can physically accommodate clients who use wheel- chairs or have other mobility impairments as well as clients with visual or hearing impairments.

able. Only 7% had a line item in their budgets for interpreters, and only one program was aware of funding available from other agencies to pay for interpreters. These statistics indicate a severe lack of understanding of what accessibility means when serving clients who have visual or hearing impairments.

Policies on Medications

Many publicly funded programs adhere to a drug-free approach to treatment and recovery. The California Department of Alcohol and Drug Programs defines a drug-free environment as one which ensures that nonprescribed psychoactive or mood-altering drugs are not used. The Department further states, "Only prescribed medications, which are for life-sustaining purposes or which are conducive to an individual's recovery process, may be used. . . . Persons who are under the care and supervision of a physician and taking prescribed or licit nonprescribed medications may . . . participate. . . . Should a program have a policy which prohibits the use of medication, other than for life-sustaining purposes, the program shall have a written policy for referring individuals to an appropriate program" (California Department of Alcohol and Drug Programs, 1984). Many local programs take this to mean no medications can be used by clients in programs licensed by the state. This is not the case; such a decision is left to individual programs with regards to *life-sustaining* medications. Further clarification is needed in defining a life-sustaining medication.

Only 65 individuals (0.31% of the total client load seen by all respondents) were known to require psychoactive medication to manage some aspect of their disabilities. However, 115 individuals were known to have been unserved during the most recent reporting year because they required medications. Twice as many potential clients who required medications were turned away as were served, apparently without being referred to an appropriate program–quite possibly because few, if any, publicly-funded appropriate programs exist. The most common referrals given to such clients were mental health programs, independent living centers and hospitals. However, independent living centers in the three counties surveyed do not provide alcohol or drug services; mental health programs are appropriate only if the client truly has a dual diagnosis. Hospitals may not be the preferred treatment modality for the economic and social-ization reasons mentioned above.

Regarding specifics about their policies on medications, 23% of respondents indicated they have policies of not accepting anyone who requires medications, 40% allowed some prescribed medica-tions, and 43% made individual client assessments regarding me-dication. Staff members dispensed all medications in 37% of pro-grams and psychoactive medications in 7%. Clients were responsible for their own medications in 43% of programs (see Figure 5). Although some medications required by people with disabilities are not accepted at up to 50% of alcohol and drug treatment programs, medications appear not to be problematic for the other half. Why, then, are the fears around prescribed medica-tions so great and the services so few for those who require them?

Outreach

One reason offered by alcohol and drug programs for not serving clients with disabilities was that they are never contacted by such clients. Where alcohol and drug programs conduct their outreach answers why this may be so. Respondents reported they regularly provide outreach to the following facilities:

- Department of Rehabilitation   37%
- Independent living centers   20%
- Disability Services Associations   10%
- Physicians who treat patients with disabilities   7%
- Disabled Students Services at local colleges and universities   0%
- No outreach to disability service agencies   17%

Obviously, very little outreach is directed specifically toward potential clients with disabilities. Not surprisingly, no particularly successful outreach strategies could be reported, although one pro-gram indicated it makes home visits and another provides trans-portation to its facility. Responses to outreach efforts were reported as mixed, ranging from minimal to excellent. The one program that had conducted what it considered substantial outreach had served several clients with disabilities.

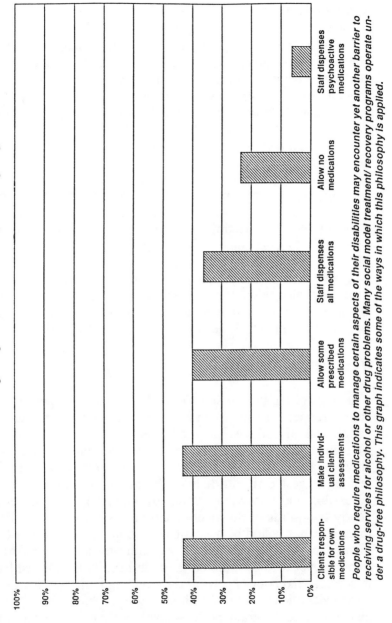

FIGURE 5. Policies Regarding Medications in Alcohol and Drug Programs

People who require medications to manage certain aspects of their disabilities may encounter yet another barrier to receiving services for alcohol or other drug problems. Many social model treatment/ recovery programs operate under a drug-free philosophy. This graph indicates some of the ways in which this philosophy is applied.

Attitudinal Barriers

Reactions among disability service professionals to the reasons offered by alcohol and drug programs for not serving clients with disabilities ranged from amusement to indignation: "Who ever has enough money?" "Why are so many people turned away because they need medications when so few programs have policies restricting them?" "Never been contacted and do nothing to change that!" "Of course, it requires extra work; that shows how little experience they have with our clients."

While no program indicated that staff awkwardness with clients with disabilities was a major obstacle, reactions from alcohol and drug providers in feedback meetings were more revealing. Statements during such meetings included: "Clients get real uncomfortable when there is somebody with a bad disability around," and "It's real hard to do the recreational things we do in a social model program when one of the people is blind or in a wheelchair." One participant also raised the question of how diligent county alcohol and drug program administrators are in applying accessibility requirements to new facilities funded within their counties.

Hope and Encouragement

In spite of the lack of services to date, 87% of respondents were at least moderately interested in improving or enhancing services to people with disabilities. They indicated the following needs (Figure 6): sign language interpreters, braille or audio-taped materials, sensitivity training for staff, and minor renovations of facilities. These results suggest that with half of the programs already physically accessible, and minor renovations by another 10% of respondents, nearly two-thirds of the alcohol and drug service systems in these three counties would be accessible to people with mobility impairments. The 43% of respondents who indicated a need for sensitivity training appear to be more on target in identifying the real barriers to service. Sixty-seven percent were willing to discuss their experiences with clients with disabilities at greater length, and 77% were available to cross-train professionals in disability services about alcohol and drug issues.

FIGURE 6. Identified Needs to Improve or Enhance Alcohol and Drug Services for People with Disabilities

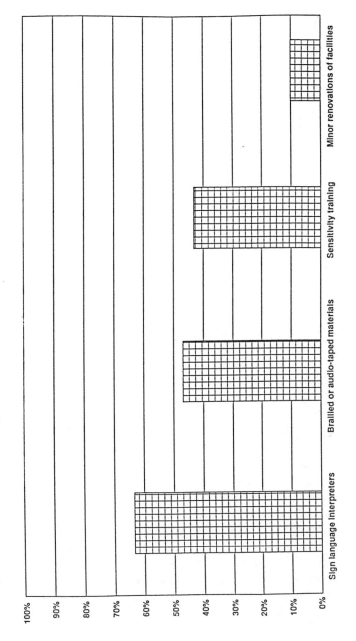

Alcohol and drug programs which have improving or enhancing services to people with disabilities as a moderate to top priority identifed the needs indicated in this graph.

DISABILITY SERVICE AGENCY SURVEYS

The disability organizations surveyed through the Bay Area Project were those recognized as providing services to or being concerned about adults with mobility, visual or hearing impairments in the three counties. Agencies that provide services on a more regional basis were also surveyed.

The decision to focus on people with mobility, visual or hearing impairments developed from two perceptions. The first was that while concerns with this population are complicated enough, issues surrounding alcohol and drug problems among people with mental or developmental disabilities are infinitely more complex. The decision was to begin with what can, in some respects, be described as people with *simpler* disabilities and then to build on this experience. A second contributing factor to this decision was the premise that from the grassroots level to the state level, advocates for those with mental and developmental disabilities are well organized and, in the case of mental health, have already begun to address the issue of dual diagnosis among that constituency.

The Institute on Alcohol, Drugs and Disability, through a contract with the California Department of Alcohol and Drug Programs, included the issue of alcohol and drug problems among people with motor, sensory, mental and developmental disabilities in its California Alcohol, Drug, and Disability Study (CALADDS). In addition, participants in task forces convened through Phase II of the Bay Area Project incorporated issues around persons with developmental disabilities, persons with dual diagnoses, and persons with traumatic brain injuries.

A four-page, 45-item survey for disability service agencies was developed by the Bay Area Project Director in consultation with the three members from the IADD Board of Directors who served as the Project Steering Committee. Input was again obtained from staff members of an alcohol program and the cosponsoring independent living center (ILC) as well as from Project funding sources. Introductory letters launching the Bay Area Project were distributed in January, 1988. Surveys, along with cover letters cosigned by both sponsors of the Bay Area Project, were sent during the first week of March to 138 programs recognized as providing services to people with disabilities. Reminder letters and duplicate surveys were sent three weeks later. By the end of April, 74 programs had returned completed surveys, for a response rate of 54%.

Of the 74 respondents, some indicated more than one option within many of the data items. Others did not respond to certain items. Therefore, the percentages listed below rarely total 100% for any one item. The percentages reflect the proportion of responses per item in relation to the entire 74 respondents.

Survey Findings

Again with this survey, we wanted to determine how much attention had been given to alcohol and drug issues within disability agencies based on the kinds of training provided to staff members. Figure 7 shows the percent of disability service staff members who received training in the last year in the following areas: working with people with AIDS, alcohol and drug problem identification and treatment, working with families, working with depressed or suicidal clients, sexuality and disability, avoiding overinvolvement with clients and potential burnout, child abuse, health promotion, advocacy skills, and battered spouses. Although it is encouraging to see that those agencies providing staff training have offered alcohol and drug sessions, only about one-third of respondents seemed to encourage staff training at all.

Service Statistics

Respondents from the three counties plus regional services in San Francisco and Santa Clara counties reported serving 35,134 clients during the most recent reporting year with the following disabilities:

• Mobility impairments	9,247
• Visual impairments	6,339
• Hearing impairments	2,204
• A combination of impairments	5,227
• Other kinds of (undesignated) disabilities	12,117

Department of Rehabilitation guidelines suggest that 15% of the 2,097,563 people or 314,634 individuals, in the three counties

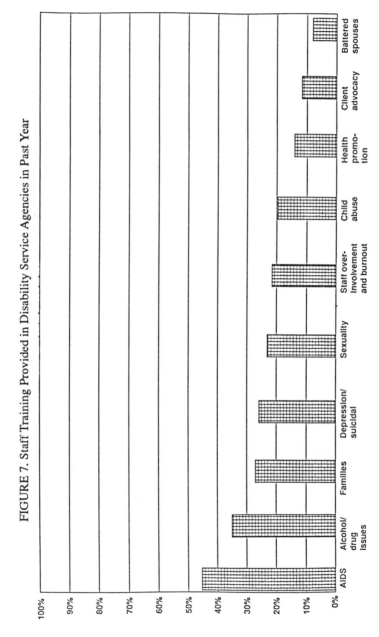

FIGURE 7. Staff Training Provided in Disability Service Agencies in Past Year

The relative importance of issues can sometimes be evaluated by the attention those issues receive in an agency. This graph depicts the percentages of disability services that provided staff training on certain client issues during the past year.

would have a disability of some sort. Thus, the agencies that responded to the Bay Area Project survey saw approximately 11% of the population with disabilities in the three counties.

When asked to estimate the prevalence of alcohol and drug problems among their clients, disability service agencies offered percentages ranging from 0.07% to 70%. The average estimate was 16%, but 35% of respondents had no idea. This wide range indicates a lack of knowledge about the alcohol or drug using behavior of clients. However, even using the 16% estimate suggests that 5,621 clients of disability service agencies surveyed are likely to have problems with alcohol or other drugs. However, only 334 individuals with disabilities were served by alcohol and drug agencies responding to the Bay Area Project survey. That represents less than 0.6% of the number estimated to be in need of such services. A more detailed question about the involvement of clients with alcohol or drugs categorized by type of impairment yielded estimates ranging from about 23% to just over 50% (see Figure 8). Again, nowhere near that number of clients were seen by the alcohol and drug programs that responded to the survey.

Identifying Problems

Completion of an Assessment Checklist of information frequently used to identify alcohol or drug problems during an intake process provided insight into why disability service agencies were unable to estimate the prevalence of such problems among their clients. They are not asking the questions that allow identification and assessment of these problems (Figure 9). Only 38% ask clients about alcohol or other drug use at all, and only 17% do so thoroughly. One reason offered by many for not asking the questions was: "If you don't ask, you don't know; then you don't have to respond to an identified need."

Figure 10 lists the percent of respondents who took specific actions when such problems were identified among clients: referred to community-based alcohol and drug programs, Alcoholics Anonymous or Narcotics Anonymous, counseling, hospital treatment programs, alcohol and other drug specialists on staff. Interestingly, six percent were not sure how to respond.

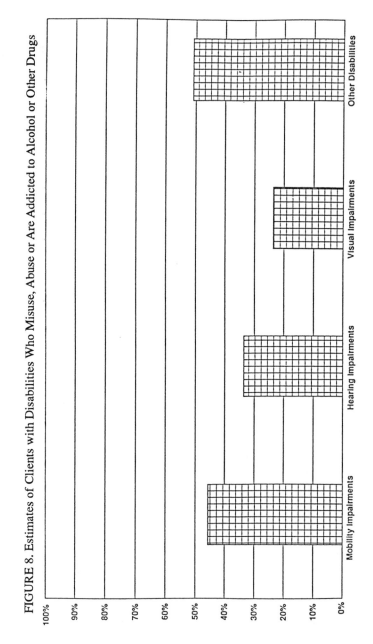

FIGURE 8. Estimates of Clients with Disabilities Who Misuse, Abuse or Are Addicted to Alcohol or Other Drugs

Estimates of alcohol or drug involvement among clients of disability service agencies vary widely. This figure indicates the average percentages of their clients that agencies believe misuse, abuse or are addicted to alcohol or other drugs (both illicit and prescription).

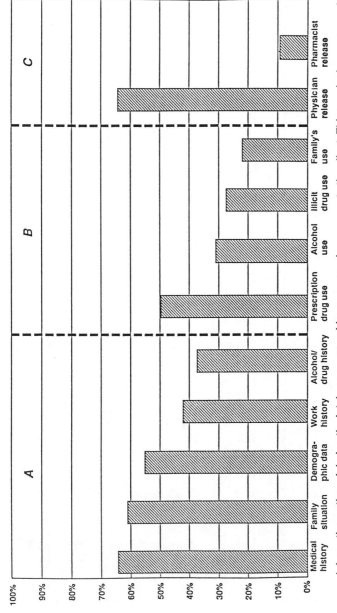

FIGURE 9. Alcohol and Drug Assessment During Intake Process

Information gathered during the intake process guides an agency's response to the client. This graph shows some of the data collected and indicates that only about one-third of disability service agencies routinely ask about alcohol and drug use during the intake process. Compilation of this and other data suggests that only 17 percent of agencies conduct an in-depth assessment of alcohol and drug use during intake.

FIGURE 10. Responses by Disability Agencies to Alcohol and Drug Problems Identified or Suspected Among Clients

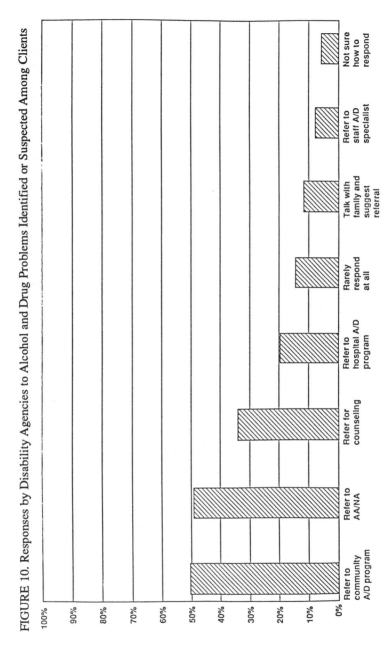

Responses to identified or suspected problems with alcohol, illicit drugs or prescription medications by service providers are significant. This graphs shows what percentages of agencies responded in a variety of ways.

Prescription Drugs

Estimates of clients suspected of misusing, abusing, or being addicted to their prescription medications ranged from one percent to 50% with the average estimate at 15%. Sixty-two percent of respondents had no idea how many clients might have such problems with medications, and two suggested the addictions were necessary. Responding organizations reacted in the following ways to such suspicions:

- Expressed concern to the client, suggested referral
  to alcohol or drug treatment   42%
- Discussed with another staff member   27%
- Rarely addressed the issue   14%
- Consulted with alcohol or drug counselor or agency   14%
- Expressed concern to family of client, suggested referral
  to alcohol or drug treatment   12%

Although the reactions to such suspicions were not especially assertive, many disability service providers profess that prescription drugs are gateway drugs of abuse for their clients and that physicians are the gatekeepers. Those with an understanding of alcohol and drug issues stress the need for physician education regarding addictions, transcending disabilities, and the need for social supports by people with disabilities.

The belief of some that given the many other difficulties in their lives, alcohol or drug problems should be of little concern to people with disabilities was addressed in the survey. Respondents reported noticing the following behaviors among disability service providers regarding alcohol and drug problems:

- Viewing alcohol and drug misuse or abuse
  as a minor issue for people with disabilities   20%
- Reluctance to address such problems   15%
- Working with clients at times when clients are under
  the influence   9%
- Allaying family concerns about client's use of alcohol
  or drugs   8%
- Helping clients to obtain alcohol or drugs   4%

Although these negative enabling behaviors were noticed in small numbers, they are significant. Reports of disability professionals inappropriately using alcohol and other drugs and, therefore, not seeing such use as problematic for their clients, were not uncommon.

Respondents were also asked whether people with disabilities are best served in special or mainstream programs. Respondents indicated preferences for the following kinds of alcohol or drug treatment and recovery programs for people with disabilities:

- Alcoholics Anonymous or Narcotics Anonymous   31%
- Alcohol and drug component within disability service
  agency   22%
- Special treatment or recovery center for people
  with disabilities   20%
- Outpatient or nonresidential alcohol and drug counseling
  program   20%
- Hospital program that treats the individual and family 15%
- Community residential program that focuses
  on the individual's lifestyle   15%

While slight preferences were shown for programs within disability service agencies or specifically for people with disabilities, the narrow range and low response rates also suggested an insufficient understanding of modalities–other than AA and NA–to make a determination.

In spite of their lack of knowledge or understanding about the issue, 42% of respondents were willing to discuss the issue of alcohol and drug problems among people with disabilities with Bay Area Project staff. Thirty-four percent had staff members who were available to train alcohol and drug service providers on accessibility and sensitivity issues.

Training Needs

During feedback meetings, professionals from each field were asked to identify training needs for themselves and for the other fields based on survey data. Training needs identified by alcohol and drug professionals during feedback meetings included:

- Dealing with clients' discomfort and distraction when another client has a disability; what is the appropriate way of acknowledging what no one is addressing; how can staff confront the group about its using the disability as a diversion; why the discomfort should be addressed as a group issue that is about life
- Reaching out effectively to disability agencies and people with disabilities
- Understanding deaf culture and differing needs of deaf clients
- Understanding prescribed medication requirements
- Insuring safety in emergency situations
- Estimating additional costs of accommodations so they can be included in budgeting process, and creative (and less costly) accommodation methods
- Finding help and resources to work with clients with disabilities
- Adapting recreational activities
- Recruiting program volunteers who have disabilities
- Understanding why mainstreaming is essential; why people with disabilities must rehabilitate in social settings since they will be living in social settings
- Understanding that recovery, transcendence of disability and independence are all variations on the same concept and goal for clients

Training needs identified by disability professionals included:

- Identifying and assessing potential and actual problems without losing the client
- Learning prevention issues, including how alcohol and other drugs can contribute to the acquisition of disabilities and how drinking and using behavior may need to change after acquiring a disability
- Overcoming the fear and dealing with the realization that recognizing alcohol and drug problems among clients could and

would put an added burden on an already overburdened system

- Understanding modalities of treatment and recovery and how to determine which is best for which clients
- Responding to abuse when it involves required medications
- Learning about alternative pain management techniques that do not require medications
- Responding appropriately when the client uses the disability to avoid getting into treatment
- Understanding that recovery, transcendence of disability, and independence are all variations on the same concept and goal for clients.

BAY AREA PROJECT–PHASE II

The Alcohol, Drugs, and Disabilities: Creating Connected Services Conference convened by the Bay Area Project in October, 1988, offered a starting point for such joint efforts. Momentum generated at the conference led to the creation of Phase II of the Bay Area Project. Phase II provided opportunities for service providers in Bay Area counties to work together and address the issue of alcohol and other drug problems among people with disabilities. Questions such as the following were raised during this process:

- Where should services be located? In disability agencies? In alcohol or drug facilities? In separate quarters?
- If in disability agencies, should there be alcohol and drug specialists on staff, or should alcohol and drug program staff come to them?
- If in alcohol and drug programs, do all facilities have to be totally accessible to people with all kinds of disabilities?
- If not, which programs would specialize in what services?
- What resources are needed to provide services?
- What funding sources are available for these resources?
- Will new resources have to be created or can existing ones be reallocated?

- Should counties work separately or does regional coordination of services make sense?

Activities, including testifying at public planning hearings, convening community forums, providing extensive cross-training efforts, conducting accessibility surveys, investigating the feasibility of regional funding, and questioning licensing requirements grew from the second phase of the Bay Area Project.

CALIFORNIA ALCOHOL, DRUG, AND DISABILITY STUDY (CALADDS)

Just as IADD was getting results back from its Bay Area surveys in early 1988, the California Department of Alcohol and Drug Programs issued a request for proposals "to make an assessment of the degree to which the needs of the alcoholic and drug abusing target population (people with disabilities in California) are not being met and to reach conclusions as to why those needs are not being met."

IADD was awarded that contract with a proposal based on replication and expansion of the Bay Area Project's survey of disability service agencies. The Department of Alcohol and Drug Programs was already in the process of "conducting a survey of non-medical alcohol and drug programs to determine the level of services to the disabled community." Launched in July, 1988, under the direction of John de Miranda, alcohol program consultant and former member of the IADD board of directors, the California Alcohol, Drug and Disability Study (CALADDS) also involved Linda Cherry, Olin Fortney, Marguerite Loya, Barbara Ludwig, Cheryl Davis, and Larry Brewster from the World Institute on Disability. CALADDS included the following components:

- Surveys of agencies that serve people with mobility, visual, and hearing impairments throughout California
- Surveys of a sample of individual clients from representative agencies listed above
- Surveys of agencies that serve people with mental health needs or with developmental disabilities to establish a baseline

of agency knowledge about the alcohol and drug problems of
these populations
- Surveys of homeless people with disabilities who may not be
involved with the disability service system

Few findings from the statewide CALADDS surveys were surprising to project team members. For the most part, they reiterated
the results of the Bay Area Project conducted in three counties and
validated the experiences of all team members in searching for
accessible alcohol and drug services. The final report for the study
was prepared by the director, John de Miranda, and issued in late
1989. It included a comprehensive set of recommendations that
were accepted by the California Department of Alcohol and Drug
Programs as guidelines for improving services for people with disabilities.

Recommendations

The unifying, global policy recommendation was that the
California Department of Alcohol and Drug Programs (ADP) declare persons with disabilities a special population at risk for alcohol and other drug-related problems requiring a variety of remedial
measures to assure access to treatment, recovery and prevention
services. To underscore the need for this policy initiative, and because of the multidisciplinary nature of the problem, de Miranda
wrote, ADP should request that the Governor create an intergovern-
mental commission (not to exceed a three-year lifespan). The
charge to this commission would be to develop and implement
strategies and initiatives that will increase access to services
through interdepartmental cooperation. Members of this commission should include the directors of the following state departments:
Alcohol and Drug Programs, Developmental Services, Social Services, Rehabilitation, Mental Health and Health Services.

Policy recommendations in the following categories were also
included in the CALADDS final report: access to care, education
and training, research and demonstration projects, agency coordination, funding, and visibility and symbolism. No attempt was made
to prioritize the recommendations in these categories which follow.

Access to Care

1. County alcohol and drug administrators (by California law, alcohol and drug services are determined at the county level to reflect local needs) should require that all startup and relocated programs make substantial effort to be fully accessible to people with orthopedic disabilities. Substantial savings can be realized by implementing accessibility features during the design and startup phase of program development, as opposed to retrofitting facilities at a later date.

2. County alcohol and drug administrators should develop and implement or update plans to modify existing program facilities to comply with Section 504 of the Rehabilitation Act of 1973.

3. County alcohol and drug program administrators should include in their annual county alcohol and drug plans a description of efforts to reach out to and include the disabled community in the annual public hearing process.

4. ADP should review the implementation of its policy regarding life-sustaining medications and recovery services, and provide clarification to service providers if deemed necessary.

5. Strategies for providing accessibility support (i.e., sign language interpreters, transportation, etc.) to 12-step programs should be explored.

6. Efforts should be made to develop recovery materials that are appropriate, meaningful, and accessible to program participants who have cognitive impairments or who have limited reading comprehension skills.

7. Accessible prevention materials targeted at adults and children should be developed. Environmental prevention materials that address special populations should always include material regarding people with disabilities.

8. Recognizing that not all programs may be able to comply with program accessibility regulations, ADP should develop a policy of sanctions for programs that are found to be consistently out of compliance with the Department's accessibility regulations and program standards. These sanctions should include contract terminations.

9. The prevention resource centers operated by the Departments

of Alcohol and Drug Programs and Education should make a special effort to provide information and materials relevant to adults and youth with disabilities.

Education and Training

1. All alcohol or drug counseling certification programs (for individuals or programs) should include a disability awareness component.

2. The alcohol and drug service field should take affirmative action to develop alcohol and drug training and prevention materials for use in disability service agencies throughout the state.

3. ADP should establish as one of its goals to train all alcohol and drug service providers in disability issues and to provide technical assistance in removing barriers to services.

4. Mechanisms should be developed to encourage and support disability service staff who wish to attend alcohol and drug training opportunities (i.e., conferences, summer schools, certificate programs, etc.).

Research and Demonstration Projects

1. The feasibility of regional services demonstration projects should be explored to develop mechanisms to facilitate multiple-county funding of services for people with disabilities. Few counties can afford to develop a full array of special services for all special populations. Inter-county cooperation in the creation of regional programming holds promise as a remediation strategy. However, the massive coordination and planning problems of multiple-county programs could probably be best addressed through a series of demonstration projects.

2. ADP should encourage efforts to explore program models to address alcohol and other drug problems among people with developmental disabilities, learning disabilities, and other cognitive impairments.

3. ADP should encourage efforts to develop a model campus-based alcohol, drug and disability prevention and recovery pilot program through a disabled student service office.

4. One-day regional forums should be developed throughout the state to disseminate CALADDS information, assist in the development of local linkages, and underscore ADP's commitment to its policy initiative.

5. Resources should be developed for a high-level two- to three-day "think tank" to provide input into and feedback about CALADDS recommendations. Such an event would pull together leaders from a variety of fields to interact and assist ADP in implementing its policy initiative.

Agency Coordination

1. Each county alcohol and drug administrator should designate a county staff person to coordinate services and information regarding access to services, and to serve as the chief liaison between state agencies, the alcohol and drug services system, and the community of persons with disabilities.

2. Efforts should be made to facilitate the formation of local task forces, made up of participants from both the disability service and alcohol and drug fields, to improve coordination and accessibility of services.

3. County alcohol and drug administrators should be encouraged to develop consultative relationships with local disability service agencies (especially independent living centers) to assist in assessing the accessibility of alcohol and drug service providers and providing technical assistance in barrier removal.

Funding

1. Use of one time federal or state funding should be explored for designation to capital accessibility enhancement and staff training for disability awareness and sensitivity. Where prohibitions against capital expenditures exist, efforts should be made to overcome or waive such prohibitions.

2. ADP should explore mechanisms for funding that will be utilized to remove barriers to services and to train alcohol and drug staff and fund monitoring and enforcement mechanisms.

3. In cases where contracts are canceled because of noncom-

pliance with accessibility regulations, counties should be encouraged to earmark such funds for affirmative remediation efforts among remaining contractors and special new programs targeted at people with disabilities.

Visibility and Symbolism

1. County alcohol and drug program administrators should actively recruit people with disabilities to serve as county staff and to serve on county alcohol and drug advisory boards, as well as the informal task forces and committees that are formed from time to time.

2. As with other special populations, people with disabilities should be recognized as being entitled to choose culturally specific programs. The availability of such programs should not have the effect of excluding people with disabilities from mainstream programs.

3. Prevention materials and activities should reflect the recognition that individuals with disabilities and individuals with chronic pain are at high risk for developing alcohol and drug problems.

4. ADP should encourage and support organizations that serve to educate the public about the special needs of people with disabilities who also have alcohol and other drug problems.

Since CALADDS was commissioned by the Department of Alcohol and Drug Programs to look at its own system, the above recommendations suggest changes in that particular system. Much of IADD's subsequent work has involved efforts to achieve complementary changes in the disability service system. Significant among those changes would be systematic education and training of service providers on identifying and assessing alcohol and drug problems among their clients with disabilities and referring them to appropriate alcohol or drug services.

CONCLUSIONS

The obvious conclusion to be drawn from the work to date of the Institute on Alcohol, Drugs and Disability is that people with both disabilities and alcohol or drug problems are a neglected population. There is tremendous avoidance of responsibility as well as a lack of understanding of the issues and possible approaches.

The work of IADD, however, seems to have opened doors for both fields to the notion that independent living and productivity are compromised, if not impossible, for anyone who is dependent upon chemicals. Confronting clients about their dependence does not jeopardize their rights to choose. Instead, addiction removes the right to choose. Recovery restores the ability to make life choices. Recovery and transcending disability are variations on the same concept and goal for clients.

Perhaps it is a question of rights. Does someone with a disability have the right to be confronted about their alcohol or drug use? Do they have the right to be held accountable for their behavior? Do they have the right to professional help when they want to change that behavior? Do they have the right to share their hope, strength and experience with peers? Do they have the right to alternative highs that bring joy to life? If so, service providers from both the disability field and the alcohol and drug field must work together. They must determine what treatment and recovery approaches are most feasible for people with various disabilities. They must make hard decisions about generating, allocating and reallocating resources. They must cooperate in advocating for systems changes that will ensure continued services.

REFERENCE

California Department of Alcohol and Drug Programs (1984). *Standards for Direct Alcohol Program Services.* Sacramento, California.

APPENDIX

IADD Publications for Outreach, Education and Prevention

In addition to the work it has accomplished through survey research and coalition building, IADD has developed a variety of publications dedicated to its mission of identifying and remediating alcohol and other drug problems among people with disabilities.

The Seed

Since it was established as one of the early IADD activities, the newsletter *The Seed* has evolved into the chronicle of information about alcohol and other drug problems among people with disabilities in California. In addition to reporting on the work of IADD, the newsletter accepts contributions from other organizations and individuals concerned with the issue. Submissions for the quarterly publication should be addressed to IADD, P.O. Box 7044, San Mateo, CA 94403. Tax-deductible donations to IADD are used to support publication of *The Seed*.

Accessibility Guidelines

An introduction to accommodating clients with disabilities is provided through IADD's *BEYOND RAMPS: A Guide to Making Alcohol and Drug Programs Accessible*. Copies of this publication are available for $1.50 each plus postage and handling through the address above.

Prevention Materials

With a mini-grant from the Alameda County Department of Alcohol and Drug Programs, IADD developed education and prevention literature that is accessible to young people who are blind or deaf. Limited copies of *THE GOOD LIFE: A Smart Choice* are available on audio tape for $2.00 each plus postage and handling or as an illustrated booklet written in simple English for $1.50 through the address above.

Bay Area Project Report

Limited copies of the complete report of the surveys conducted through Phase I of the Bay Area Project on Disabilities and Chemical Dependency are also available for $3.00 each plus postage and handling.

California Alcohol, Drug, and Disability Study

Copies of the California Alcohol, Drug, and Disability Study (CA-LADDS) are available. The executive summary is $2 plus postage and handling. Volume I includes summaries of the surveys and recommendations and is $10. Volume II contains all data charts and is also $10 plus postage and handling.

Literature Review

As part of the CALADDS project, IADD developed a comprehensive review of the literature concerning alcohol, drugs and disability. This review is available for $5 plus postage and handling.

IADD publications can be requested by writing to P.O. Box 7044, San Mateo, CA 94403.

Chapter 14

Comprehensive Treatment of Addictive Families

Stephen E. Schlesinger, PhD
Lawrence K. Horberg, PhD

Addictions tax families heavily. Social circles shrink, economic and emotional security are threatened, psychological growth is stymied, and relationships among family members are strained. The longer the problems persist, the greater the damage. There are many approaches to family treatment of addiction (for a discussion, please see Schlesinger, 1988 and Schlesinger and Gillick, 1989). This chapter describes a practical approach to treating addictive families, designed to help them repair the damage, create more satisfying lives, and prevent long-lasting deleterious effects, commonly associated with codependency and which affect children of addicts.

This approach is grounded in a developmental model of family recovery which was devised to meet the needs of members of this population while, at the same time, taking into account their high level of diversity.

This chapter summarizes four points which highlight this approach. Then it considers the process of treatment in more detail. At the end of the chapter, several considerations are discussed concerning the application of this approach to families in which one or more members have a disability.

HIGHLIGHTS OF THE APPROACH

First, the approach focuses on engaging all interested family members in a journey from chaos to family health. It takes issue with those approaches which view the family as an instrument to coerce the addict into recovery, with those which ignore the addiction, and with those which ignore the family's needs.

Second, for many families, the journey begins in a state of exasperation, hopelessness and helplessness. It proceeds through a period of experimentation and effort. The journey reaches a state in which family members feel hopeful about, in charge of, and competent to handle their lives.

Third, the approach focuses on helping family members confront the addiction itself by engaging in a stepwise process of withdrawing from destructive experiences related to addiction. Setting limits is a crucial part of the process but is not a method of controlling the addict. Limits are set both to protect the family and to communicate the family's healthy resolve.

Fourth, there are specific actions and foci of attention required for successful recovery. The approach lays out these developmental tasks in logical order. A series of exercises has been developed to help guide family members through these tasks.

THE PROCESS OF TREATMENT

Recovery is defined as the process of repairing the damage done by the addiction and creating more satisfying lives. The process is organized into four areas of developmental tasks which flow from the last of the four points highlighted above. In *Getting Started*, family members develop a realistic basis for hope that solutions to their problems are possible to devise and that they can solve their problems. In part, this process arises from helping family members define those problems in terms which promote action.

Many families decide that they will take action on their problems–including coming for professional help–at a point at which they are depleted emotionally, and frequently physically. It is important, therefore, to help family members refocus their attention on their own lives, apart from the addict, in order that they might fortify themselves for the tasks of recovery. Therefore, in the second task area, *Strengthening the Family*, family members learn to take better care of themselves, live fuller lives and develop the supportive relationships they will need in order to face the addiction once again.

Once they feel stronger, family members can face the third task area, *Confronting the Addiction*. This involves focusing on what generally is termed enabling. Specifically, this means learning which family resources and benefits support destructive behaviors and learning both how to set limits for self-protection and how to avoid inadvertently supporting an addiction.

When family members have withdrawn from the poisonous experiences so often associated with chaotic behavior, they are ready to focus their attention on the fourth area, *Flourishing as a Family*. This involves, generally, replacing a survivor mentality with a flourishing mentality as the first step in helping relatives develop and live healthy, nonchaotic lives. Among other things at this point in recovery, family members learn to let go of the lingering effects of trauma occasioned by living with an addict, navigate some common pitfalls in recovery, and build healthy communication patterns.

Let us return now to consider the four developmental task areas in some detail. This approach to treatment uses a number of different tools to engage and treat families, some the same as others (e.g., self-help groups) and some different. We will focus here on the unique parts this approach may contribute to family treatment. Examples and exercises to apply this approach are elaborated in Schlesinger and Horberg (1988).

GETTING STARTED

How does one engage, in treatment, a family which may, among other things, feel hopeless and helpless in their situation, may be despairing, may blame itself for the addict's behavior, may be ignoring its own pain, and may have neglected the safety, comfort and well-being of its members? This is a type of family in which there is a lot of motion–energy expended randomly in reaction to the chaos which an addiction creates, but little movement–energy expended *pro*actively in healthy and productive directions. As a first step in helping family members make sense of the pain they feel and to work past it, a metaphor is presented. This metaphor casts recovery as a journey, and it helps dispel the notion that recovery is an event. It suggests that family members who recover successfully move through three regions, the 3 E's: Exasperation, Effort, and Empowerment.

Recovery as a Journey

In Region I, chaos is a fact of everyday life. Family members feel confused, exhausted, scared, and extremely pessimistic about their ability to influence their futures. It is a state of fragmentation in which family members feel Exasperated, with little idea of what they can do to end their pain.

One problem with being consumed with an addiction–either one's own or one's relative's–is that devotion to chaos stunts personal growth. In the process of diverting one's attention from growth to destructive behaviors, one misses many opportunities to grow. It is not uncommon, for example, for adult addicts who have drug use histories dating to childhood or adolescence to characterize one aspect of recovery as "growing up." Family members affected by addictions often need a chance to begin to grow, and the first step in this process often is a period of exploration and experimentation to make up for lost experiences. Region II is a period of unrelenting Effort, often in what family members see as a gray world, in which they begin to do things which are different (or to do old things in new ways), without a clear idea of where they will lead. It is a period which can be taxing in that family members do not get a specific return for particular actions they take. It frequently strains the family's resolve to get better.

In Region III, family members develop a sense of purpose and become meaningfully involved in many aspects of their lives. They feel alive and lively, competent to face and solve problems which come up and eager to make commitments to healthy activities and relationships. They feel a sense of Empowerment. Whereas Region I was a period of fragmentation, Region III is one of integration.

An irony presents itself in the midst of this journey. Recovery really begins when family members decide, in Region I, that they will do *whatever it takes* to end their pain. It is in this way that they pass into Region II. However, in Region II family members find the effort required rather tedious. This results, in part, from the lack of direction people often feel in Region II. Nevertheless, it is important for people to make decisions and take constructive actions in Region II, even if they seem pointless in the absence of the structure and hopefulness they achieve once they enter Region III. To remedy this problem, it is helpful for family members to try to answer four basic questions as they make decisions along the way. The questions are as follows:

Question 1:	*What kind of experience do I want right now?*
Question 2:	*What choices or actions would I admire in myself in this situation?*
Question 3:	*What strengths do I have that would be valuable in this situation?*
Question 4:	*What do I feel right now?*

These four questions can be helpful in providing a temporary framework within which people can stop and make considered decisions in their journey to health, and family members are encouraged to write them down (or memorize them) and to answer them in as many circumstances during the day as may be required. Use of the four questions allows family members to see themselves taking charge of their lives, and for some this may have followed a substantial period in which they felt helpless and paralyzed.

One measure of progress in recovery can be the changing themes in the answers to the four questions as family members move through the three regions. A helpful table depicting these themes is included below as Table 1.

Defining the Problem

The next step in Getting Started is to help family members define their problems concretely and in terms which promote family action. This can be conceptualized as a five-step process, each part of which defines an exercise for family members. The steps are as follows:

Step 1:	Identifying Family Problems
Step 2:	Separating Facts from Opinions

Step 3:   Identifying Facts Related to Addiction
Step 4:   Identifying Feelings Associated with Those Facts
Step 5:   Identifying Family Strengths

The process of helping family members define their problems can be quite instructive. It is helpful in Step 3, for example, for family members to see that there may be important family problems not related to addiction. This helps them define family health more broadly than simply the absence of addictive behaviors. It is crucial, as well, for family members in Step 5 to understand clearly what their strengths are. Few families coming for treatment truly have no strengths, even though many might perceive their situations in such catastrophic terms. In many instances, family members function in different regions in different aspects of their lives. For example, an effective, dynamic corporate vice president (Region III at work) may also inadvertently support a child's cocaine use which is destroying the family (Region I at home). This person may have many strengths which will be helpful in the family's recovery, though the chaos of the addiction may obscure them from view.

It is helpful for family members to complete the definition of their problems by considering the interplay of their emotions. This can be conceptualized in outline form as a 2 (positive/negative) by 2 (addiction-related/nonaddiction related) table (Figure 1). *Positive* feelings about drugs and alcohol have to be considered because they will help broaden the family's understanding of its goals and its possible resistance to growth. For example, if an addict is amorous only when drunk, the spouse may be reluctant to have him give up alcohol or to make their sex life contingent on sobriety.

STRENGTHENING THE FAMILY

Once addiction-related and other problems have been defined, the process of setting realistic goals begins by turning attention away from the addiction and focusing on the loved ones themselves and on their lives.

Helping family members focus on their wants, abilities, commitments and good points will help them counteract the feelings of

TABLE 1. Themes of Answers to the Four Questions in Each Region

Characteristics of the Regions	Question 1 *What kind of experiences do I want right now?*	Question 2 *What choices or actions would I admire in myself in this situation?*	Question 3 *What strengths do I have that would be valuable in this situation?*	Question 4 *What do I feel right now?*
III. EMPOWERMENT Purpose and meaning Alive! and lively risk taking Commitment Involvement with others Responsibility clearly defined	*Fulfilling dreams.* A person can dream, plan to fulfill the dream and enjoy it when it comes together. Dreams are based on true understanding of needs. His sense of entitlement and sense of responsibility are realistic.	*Taking responsibility.* A person lives out his own values, takes credit for his successes, and defines ways of improving further.	*Believing in strengths.* A person feels loveable, likable and effective. He can define his strengths and count on them when taking on challenges.	*Experiencing at a deep level.* Full range of positive and negative feelings and passions. Sense of personal competence leads to a feeling of serenity.

TABLE 1 (continued)

	Safe pleasures.	*Pleasing others.*	*Groping for strengths.*	*Tentatively opening up to feelings.*
II. EFFORT Relentless effort in a grey world, without certain reward Going through the motions Surviving	Blandness and socially acceptable pleasures are all that one looks forward to. Fulfilling deep needs seems impossible.	A person gets vague satisfaction from choosing socially acceptable alternatives.	A person is able to win recognition from others but feels hollow, as if merely going through the motions or as if he is an imposter.	Deeper feelings are emerging but are difficult to define. "Is that all there is?"
I. EXASPERATION Chaos, shame, helplessness Vulnerability	*Conflict interferes with pleasures.* Needs are not understood; rarely gratified out in the open.	*Little is admired.* A person holds many conflicting standards, but only at a shallow level. He violates his most basic standards. Life is chaotic, and he perceives others as looking down on him.	*Few strengths are evident.* A person's opinion of himself swings from inferiority to superiority.	*Denying and discounting feelings.* Feelings are superficial and mainly in reaction to chaos and confusion.

From: Stephen E. Schlesinger and Lawrence K. Horberg (1988). *Taking Charge: How Families Can Climb Out of the Chaos of Addiction . . . and Flourish.* New York: Fireside Books/Simon and Schuster, pages 24-25.

FIGURE 1. 2 x 2 Table Mapping the Experiences of an Addictive Family

	ADDICTION-RELATED EXPERIENCES	EXPERIENCES FREE OF ADDICTIVE BEHAVIOR
POSITIVE EXPERIENCES	1. "Giving" only when intoxicated. 2. Generous and relaxed after a big gambling win. 3. Cleaning and organizing binge accompanies drinking. 4. Singing, dancing, being "the life of the party" with or without friends, after using cocaine and alcohol. 5. Drinking to overcome the pain of physical therapy and for "courage" during a period of consistent effort at rehabilitation. 6. Using steroids to build muscle after developing the hobby of competitive weight-lifting, to compensate for feelings of inferiority.	1. Family attends wheelchair basketball games regularly, enjoying friendship and support of other families. 2. Spouses enjoy a passionate physical relationship free of addictive behavior. 3. Quiet male sibling masters computer program that allows him to get a meaningful job. 4. Family business prospers. 5. First born daughter is very popular in school.
NEGATIVE EXPERIENCES	1. Smashing up the car, driving while under the influence. 2. Experiencing an acute toxic reaction to prescribed medication because of interactions with alcohol. 3. Being arrested after selling cocaine to other patients in a rehab hospital. 4. Repeated episodes of drunken "pity parties" with incoherent slurred diatribes against imagined enemies. 5. Failure to attend rehab appointments when "high" on pain medication. 6. Bookies appear at the family home looking for "----" in the wheelchair, to break anything that's not already broken".	1. Strained relations with the extended family, who appear to have dropped out of sight after the onset of the disability. 2. Father has rarely expressed affection to anyone in the family. 3. Two of the younger children appear to be socially withdrawn. 4. The house appears to be in a state of disrepair. 5. The dog has never been adequately trained. Housebreaking has been neglected. 6. Money is very tight.

hopelessness that bog down the family. By acknowledging areas of strengths, the family equips itself to make use of them.

Until *self*-examination begins, despair increases, the world appears to shrink. Eventually, it may seem that the only important events in the family have to do with the addiction: "Did he seem high when he came home?" "Will she overdose tonight?" "Will she even come home?"

In considering their depleted state, families focus on three areas: Living a full life, Increasing self-care activities, and Developing supportive relationships.

Living a Full Life

In this section, family members explore the relationship between living a full life and ending members' participation in family pathology. Living a full life is at the core of recovery.

To the extent that family members know which experiences they want and which they detest, which of their choices and actions make them proud and which shame them, which situations stir feelings that enrich their lives and which detract from them, they will feel the motivation to take action and leave chaos behind. To the extent they know and exercise their strengths, they will feel confident in their ability to live a full life. To the extent members are unable to answer the four questions, they will be mired in confusion.

Families vary in their determination to live a full life and maintain their values. As a result, they also differ in the way they decide when enough is enough and when to take decisive action. Of interest to therapists are the general questions: When do families act? When do they become determined to fight their way out of the exasperation of Region I?

People act at different points to tackle their problems. Decision points can be conceptualized on a continuum which has four points, ranging from relatively untraumatic to life-threatening, as follows:

a. distaste for the addict's behavior
b. public embarrassment; distaste for own behavior
c. threat to property and safety
d. endangered lives

There are two general tasks for living a full life. The first is for family members to clarify their wants, standards, strengths and feelings. The second task guides family members through an examination of some of the cognitive components of recovery. It focuses on overcoming barriers to a full life and identifies some opinions that obstruct recovery efforts and others which motivate healthy action. Table 2 describes some common barriers.

Increasing Self-Care Activities

Whereas deteriorating self-care can damage the family further, habits of self-care, vigorously maintained, provide a family with strength and a sense of dignity and well-being. These habits fall into three important areas: General health and hygiene, maintenance of safety, well-being and comfort, and management of stress. Each individual assumes some responsibility for himself in these areas, and the adults in the family assume additional responsibility to establish routines for the family.

An important aspect of self-care which frequently is neglected in addictive families concerns their abilities to manage stress. In many cases, family members equate stress management with problem solving. Although problem solving is clearly an aspect of effective stress management, constantly trying to solve unsolvable problems (e.g., someone else's addiction) merely offers the relative a chance to fail over and over again.

An alternative to this unidimensional view of stress management is to view the management of stress from the broader perspective of an individual's lifestyle. This view follows from the work of Ayala Pines and Elliott Aronson (see, for example, Pines and Aronson, 1988).

Activities to manage stress can be conceptualized along two dimensions: activity (active vs. inactive) and object of attention (toward the stressor vs. away from the stressor). If we assemble these dimensions in a 2 x 2 format, we can define four components of a stress management lifestyle. It is this conception which family members examine at this point in recovery.

Active methods which direct attention toward the stressor reduce future stress by getting directly at the source. For example, when

TABLE 2

Overcoming Barriers to a Full Life

To appreciate the fullness of one's life, to revive desirable commitments that have been cast aside, to protect existing values from the chaos of addiction and to enrich family life in new ways, some families must challenge opinions they have of themselves that inhibit bold action. We offer the items in the table "Overcoming Barriers to a Full Life" as examples of opinion changes that often help build momentum toward recovery.

Overcoming Barriers to a Full Life

Opinions That Weaken	*Opinions That Motivate*
1. I failed myself and my family, and I do not deserve to live a good life.	1. I did the best I know how to do. I want to live the best life I can. Hurting myself, holding back or being miserable will help no one. I am human and will make mistakes. For now, I'll do the next right thing.
2. There is a blight on my family. We'd better not show our faces. We are pariahs.	2. All families endure pain, shame or vulnerability at some point. There is dignity in accepting and coping with family problems. Some people may "throw stones," but others will respect what we are trying to do.
3. Our lives are awful because of the addiction. They will get better only when the addict learns how terrible he is and pays us back for our trouble. There is nothing I can do until then.	3. Our lives are what we make of them. If I am frustrated, I must want something. If I feel inadequate, there must be something I want to do better. If I feel unfulfilled, there must be something I want to accomplish. I cannot wait for the addict, I must live my life now (and help my children live their lives now). My values, my satisfactions, my problems are my responsibility.
4. My satisfaction will come when I reform the addict. Then I will have done something really important. The addict has such potential, so much more than I do! If I could be the one to help him, he would take care of me and accept my weaknesses.	4. I cannot save anyone. I have to develop my own strengths, be the best person I can be.
5. The addict is only hurting me, and that does not really matter, If he were hurting others in our family, then I would have to do something. My welfare is unimportant.	5. I will no longer permit anyone to damage me or to stop me from living a full life. I am important, every bit as important as any other member of my family.
6. I am–for the addict–the patient and loving person I myself needed all these years. To be firm right now would be harsh and cruel. It would create, for the addict, the same lousy conditions I have had to live under my whole life.	6. I want support and will seek it. I want to give support, but I can only support health. I can no longer cater to abuse. To coddle an addict is not to help him.

From: Stephen E. Schlesinger and Lawrence K. Horbert (1988). *Taking Charge: How Families Can Climb Out of the Chaos of Addiction . . . and Flourish.* New York: Fireside Books/Simon and Schuster, pages 86 and 87.

the family prohibits drunk driving among its members, it prevents worry and suffering. Successful stress reduction depends in part on effective problem solving. In this regard, it is helpful to review seven effective components of problem solving with family members. They are as follows:

1. Quickly and naturally focus attention on problems as they arise.
2. Define problems clearly to promote problem solving.
3. Talk with others to get information, support and help in organizing an approach to the problem.
4. Think of alternative solutions.
5. Take direct action by asserting self and making arrangements with others.
6. Take direct action by doing independent work.
7. Follow up and stick with routines designed to prevent problems in the future.

Inactive methods focusing attention on the stressor focus on *thinking and talking* about problems and other stressors. Family members often think of problems in a mental shorthand which does not lend itself to problem resolution. Putting thoughts into words requires that the problems be made concrete. In this regard, complaining can be helpful, and family members are encouraged to use it. Complaining is a highly underrated activity. It promotes ventilation of feelings, reorganization of thoughts, clarification of goals and wants, and identification of stressors. To move forward, families must give themselves permission to complain. When complaining replaces suffering in silence, the family is getting better.

Active methods of focusing attention away from stressors refresh the spirit and enhance self-esteem away from the family's field of battle. We emphasize that there is no way to help the addict if family members stop living, if they let themselves be consumed by the problem. To avoid this, they must include activities in their lives which help them have fun and grow. These may involve hobbies, exercise and other active activities which family members enjoy, but which do not bear directly on the addict or the addiction.

Inactive methods of focusing attention away from stressors address the erroneous notion that we must remain productive every waking moment. In fact, we also need time to *escape,* to engage in idle activities which help refresh us. These may include naps, meditation, reading a book, watching television, or anything else which allows a respite from the stress of one's life.

Balance is important in any lifestyle which is created to minimize stress. Those who spend most of their energies in one or another of the four categories of activities will be less successful in managing their stress than those who spread their activities among the four.

Developing Supportive Relationships

The third area involved in strengthening the family is developing supportive relationships. Families grow stronger as their members develop relationships with people outside the family; involvement with others does four important things. First, it strengthens personal identity. Since addiction and social isolation go hand in hand, family members are often stripped of their roles, and, therefore, stripped of their identities. When we perform our roles well, we think of ourselves as competent. Others help us maintain a stable sense of identity.

Second, involvement with others enhances positive aspects of our lives. Relationships and social contacts provide stimulation, variety, recognition, communication, closeness, attraction, intimacy, sense of purpose, useful activity, practical help, challenge and structure. Many of the best things in life occur with other people. Without contact with others, life can bebarren, empty and painful.

Third, involvement with others increases emotional support and challenge. Addicts sometimes command most of the attention in the family, interfering with the family's attempt to understand its everyday world and blinding family members to the possibility of finding support through involvement with others. Events in a chaotic family are difficult to think about and comprehend. In order to develop an understanding, family members must first put their experiences into words and describe them to others, even though at first their descriptions may sound disloyal, provocative or offensive. Without access to supportive listeners, family members can never get past the numerous dead ends in their thinking. With support, however, experiences–no matter how painful–are accepted, discussed and incorporated into the family's understanding of itself. Families can then describe their everyday lives in terms that stick.

Fourth, involvement with others increases informational support and challenge, practical knowledge that helps in problem solving or in accomplishing things. Involvement with friends and groups naturally increases our access to expertise generally.

Developing supportive relationships is crucial to family recovery. However, there are several barriers to developing supportive relationships. These include four ideas: (1) outside contacts are viewed as extremely threatening; (2) outside relationships stir up feelings of inadequacy in people who suffer from low self-esteem; (3) realizing that the addict has no right to limit your involvement in life is a critical step in recovery; and (4) some of the family's beliefs may impede the effort to develop outside relationships.

CONFRONTING THE ADDICTION

Once the family has strengthened itself and replenished its depleted emotional and physical resources, it is time for members to focus once again on the addiction. The focus is not on how the family can persuade a reluctant addict to stop his drug use or go for treatment. Rather, the focus is on how the family can extricate itself from involvements with the addict which are unhealthy for the family and which may inadvertently support the addiction.

Most support given to the addict, ranging from small favors to the continuation of relationships, is given on a voluntary basis. Yet it never seems that way. It can seem to loved ones as if they have *no control* over their own actions. The illusion that they have no control can be so powerful that the even therapist has a hard time believing otherwise.

The therapeutic goal at this point is to cut off support for addictive and other chaotic behaviors in the family safely, while selectively increasing the family's ability to support healthy patterns. Related objectives include, first, helping relatives learn which resources, actions, and decisions they *do* control and which they do *not* control. This helps weaken the illusion of control over the addict's behavior and strengthen awareness of control over members' own behavior, participation, resources, and decisions.

A second objective is to increase members' understanding of how specific forms of support often enable the addict to continue engaging in destructive behavior. Support allows the addict to escape the consequences of drug use and may even create the opportunity for abuse where it would otherwise not exist. The third objective is to increase loved ones' abilities to communicate feelings and observations related to addiction. Family members are then ready to tackle the fourth objective: with a minimum of effort and risk, withhold support for addictive behavior by setting limits.

The structure of the overall effort to confront the addiction involves guiding the family through four decisions as they cut off support for chaotic/addictive behavior:

1. *What* support to withhold;
2. *When* to withhold it;
3. *What to say* to the addict about the changes in the family; and
4. What are our *goals*?

The process of withdrawing support for addictive behavior is similar in some ways to the classical intervention techniques practiced widely in addictions treatment centers. However, as practiced, intervention has several drawbacks. First, if it does not work, there may be nothing left to try. Second, it may inadvertently set the family up to back down and to remain inconsistent in its dealings with the addict. For example, a family which devises an intervention strategy with a counselor which tells the addict, in effect, to "get well or get out" may face his resistance and then have to decide whether they really want to stick to their threat to kick him out. If not, then once again, no meant yes. Chaotic behavior is reinforced on an intermittent schedule.

An alternative is for the family to take a slower, more persistent approach in which it withholds only part of the support it provides the addict and escalates only if necessary. Family members approach their disengagement in a stepwise fashion. Limit setting is not approached as a method of controlling the addict. Loved ones learn when to limit their involvement with the addict so as to avoid unhealthy or harmful contact. It begins with an assessment of the resources controlled by the family which support addiction and proceeds to create an action plan to withhold them when certain chaotic behaviors occur.

When asked to list the resources under their control, family members often draw a blank. Over the years, they have made many decisions automatically. They may think that if they care about the addict, they cannot or should not withhold anything from him. They may feel guilty and believe that they owe him anything and everything they give. Fear may blind them to the real control they could have (e.g., "If I stop pretending, will he leave me? destroy my future? kill me?")

Resources can be described as benefits people receive as family members in good standing. Benefits can be of four different sorts: material support, effort on behalf of and attention to the addict, companionship, and confirmation or reassurance that the addict is a member of the family in good standing. In chaotic families, benefits are provided *non*contingently. Confronting the addiction is, in part, a process of making these benefits available on a contingent basis.

Decision 1: What to Withhold

Family members frequently find it difficult to identify those things which they control and which they potentially could withhold from the addict when the addict engages in self-destructive behaviors. Benefits fall into two categories: material and nonmaterial support. The most easily identified benefits typically are material. They include, for example, room and board, use of the car, money, and basic necessities. Nonmaterial support includes companionship, efforts on the addict's behalf, and personal acknowledgement or confirmation.

Decision 2: When to Withhold

Once family members have an idea of what they have available to withhold, they are ready to consider the next question: when to withhold benefits from the addict. The answer to this question is two-fold. First, family members need to identify some target behaviors which they decide are unhealthy for them and unacceptable on the part of the addict. We encourage family members to think of limit setting and enforcement in if-then (or contingent) terms. In other words, family members think of making the provision of these benefits contingent on whether the addict is acting in acceptable ways. This sets the stage for family members to identify concrete, unacceptable behaviors which then can serve as the foundation for setting limits. In the if-then formulation, family members create an action plan in which the ifs are specific behaviors and the thens are benefits to be withheld if the behaviors occur (or to be offered in the absence of those behaviors). The if-then chart which results from this process constitutes an action plan to guide the family's response to unacceptable behavior by the addict.

The second part of the answer to when to withhold is to help family members consider the stance the addict has toward his addiction at the time. Stances range from the addict being in a life or death struggle as a result of his addiction through five other stages, to being abstinent and committed to a program of recovery. Family members may learn to vary their responses to otherwise unacceptable behavior depending on which stage they believe the addict to be in. If the addict is truly in a life or death situation, for example, the family may choose to respond in a manner calculated to rescue the addict, even though at other times this may seem to support the very behavior they find unacceptable.

Having placed itself in a position to act, how then does the family talk to the addict about its decisions?

Decision 3: What to Say to the Addict

Limits are incomplete unless they are communicated to the addict. This, however, must be evaluated in terms of family members' safety. Chaotic families are at higher risk for violence, and it is important that family members not expose themselves to potential danger in talking to the addict.

We cannot tell our clients what to say. But, we suggest several guidelines to frame family members' thoughts about talking to the addict. First, we encourage them to make *simple statements* of facts, derived from their if-then charts, if possible. Second, telling the addict *one thing at a time* is most effective. Third, being *brief and to the point* is crucial. Fourth, it is most helpful if family members emphasize the positive reasons the family is going to the trouble of communicating.

It is important to discuss with family members ahead of time the fact that the addict's drug use may continue even after the family withholds support for addiction. It is crucial that the family be very clear about what their goal is in withholding support for addictive behavior. The family's goal at this point is to disengage itself from complicity–intended or not–in the addictive process so *it*, not the addict, can get better.

FLOURISHING

When family members have withdrawn themselves from unhealthy involvement with the addiction, they are ready to look ahead to creating satisfying lives for themselves. The goals in treatment at this point are to help families let go of trauma, overcome some common obstacles to progress, and see images of recovery which can act as guides until they can formulate their own.

Letting Go of Trauma

Living with the impact of addictive behaviors can be traumatic for family members. They feel a lot of pain, sometimes for extended periods of time. When they have removed themselves from the traumatic situation successfully, they must face the effects of the trauma so they can move on. For this task, family members are introduced to a three-step model process through which they can move past the impact of the trauma. It is called the 3 Rs: Retribution, Restitution, and Refuge. In step one, family members feel an acute sense of Retribution, a longing for the addict to suffer in a manner commensurate with the pain they believe he has inflicted. Making concrete the means through which this suffering would occur usually is not possible, however. At that point, family members move on to step 2, in which they hope for Restitution from the addict for their suffering. When the currency of this repayment becomes hard to define and when current needs are gratified, family members typically move on to the third step. This involves seeking Refuge, or protection, from the possible recurrence of conditions which caused pain previously. The idea of refuge is an important one. Family members need to reduce the feeling of vulnerability they sometimes feel when they tackle the job of moving forward with their recovery. The action plan they develop in the if-then chart often provides a good measure of protection for family members.

Overcoming Obstacles to Progress

There are several obstacles to progress to which it is helpful to inoculate family members. Family members who expect smooth sailing sometimes interpret what are otherwise common obstacles as major complications in treatment and signs of the failure of their efforts. We divide these obstacles into the eight categories listed below.

1. Fear of uncertainty, change, and emptiness
2. Getting over the hump
3. Losing sight of the goal
4. Getting hung up on details
5. Embarrassment
6. Counterproductive, or dysfunctional, communication
7. Blaming
8. Inertia

At this point, family members have progressed through the stages of getting started, strengthening themselves, withdrawing their support for the addiction, formulating and communicating their healthy resolve, getting past the trauma which chaotic family life left in its wake, and preparing themselves to face obstacles as they continue their recovery. Family members now need to learn to flourish.

The first step in understanding the concept of flourishing is to recognize that family recovery can have any of a variety of outcomes. Anticipating the possibilities is important if family members are to set reasonable expectations upon which to judge their progress accurately. If, for example, family members come to expect that successful family recovery can be achieved only if all members of the family get better at the same time and the family reconstitutes itself fully, many families may be disappointed and interpret their efforts as failures. Preparing families for the possibility that recovery may be represented in a variety of outcomes is another way of inoculating them and helping them anticipate potential obstacles to a realistic view of their efforts.

Recovery at this point continues with the family's focus on creating healthy, satisfying lives. To the extent that family members have developed the skills they need to handle their problems, they may be confident of their ability to continue on their own. To the extent that some of the nonaddiction-related problems identified in Getting Started remain active, family members may choose to remain in counseling in order to tackle outstanding difficulties.

FAMILIES WITH MEMBERS WHO HAVE DISABILITIES

Physical disabilities–either in the addict or in other family members–complicate the assessment and treatment planning process. The Taking Charge model provides a flexible approach to the special needs of families with members who have disabilities. For example, guilt may be intensified in a family when it considers withholding benefits from a disabled addict. In this case, the traditional all-or-nothing approach to intervention would be particularly inappropriate. In addition, there are special challenges facing an individual with a disability who is in the early stages of learning how to flourish. Therapeutic attention must be directed to overcoming physical barriers, self- pity, the sick role, and the tendency to discount the potential of handicapped addicts or family members to flourish.

SUMMARY

The purpose of our developmental model is to create tools to address the needs of addictive families: needs many families have in common and needs that are highly individual. The emphasis is on flexible application.

REFERENCES

Pines, A. and Aronson, E. (1988). *Career Burnout: Causes and Cures.* New York: Free Press.

Schlesinger, S.E. (1988). Cognitive-behavioral approaches to family treatment of addictions. In N. Epstein, S.E. Schlesinger, and W. Dryden (Eds.). *Cognitive-Behavioral Therapy with Families* (pp. 254-291). New York: Brunner/Mazel.

Schlesinger, S.E. and Gillick, J. (1989). *Stop Drinking and Start Living* (Second Ed.). Blue Ridge Summit, PA: TAB Books.

Schlesinger, S.E. and Horberg, L.K. (1988). *Taking Charge: How Families Climb Out of the Chaos of Addiction . . . and Flourish.* New York: Fireside Books/Simon and Schuster.

Chapter 15

Evaluating Treatment Services

Thomas J. Budziack, PhD

In Chapter 11, Reid Hester discussed the importance of developing individualized interventions tailored to the client. Chapter 9 described attitudes among substance abuse treatment professionals that often impede treatment individualization. The homogeneity assumption, the notion that all substance abusers have similar characteristics, together with the assumption that there is one best way to treat addictions, were described as major barriers to individualized treatment.

This chapter focuses on how rehabilitation professionals can overcome these obstacles and help arrange appropriate individualized treatment for persons with disabilities who abuse alcohol and other drugs. To be an effective referral counselor and case manager, the rehabilitation professional must be able to (1) arrange objective alcohol and other drug abuse (AODA) assessments for his or her clients; (2) evaluate the services provided by AODA treatment providers; and (3) refer clients to the type of treatment that best meets their individual needs. The first step in this process is to understand the types of AODA treatment services available in most communities.

AODA TREATMENT

Most traditional treatment programs promote 28-day inpatient treatment. This type of treatment is typically program-driven: Each day is programmed with a set of predetermined activities from early morning through the evening. In accordance with the homogeneity assumption, most treatment hours are devoted to group activities that provide the core treatment that all alcoholics and addicts are believed to require. This type of program almost invariably follows a strict Twelve-Step orientation. Procedures and approaches that are not consistent with the Twelve-Step philosophy usually are not incorporated.

Intensive outpatient programs typically involve from four to six hours of treatment activities per day for five to six days per week over a period of three to six weeks. This type of program is usually program-driven, using abbreviated versions of the treatment schedules followed in 28-day inpatient programs.

Individualized treatment programs focus on designing a program that fits the individual client. A genuinely individualized program will use a wide variety of treatment modalities and procedures which are tailored to the characteristics and needs of the individual. Treatment following a Twelve-Step orientation is usually one of the modalities available, but clients are not required to conform to Twelve-Step principles if they are not amenable.

AODA treatment is offered in a variety of settings. One of the most common is *general hospital-based AODA treatment programs.* During the early 1980s, hundreds of these programs were established by general hospitals with a declining census. National franchise-type firms aggressively promoted AODA wards as a rapid and inexpensive way to convert under-utilized hospital wings to profit centers. Hospital-based programs usually promote 28-day inpatient treatment as the preferred intervention, although many have begun to offer intensive outpatient treatment as well.

Free-standing AODA treatment programs are facilities dedicated to AODA treatment which are independent of another hospital. Most are committed to 28-day inpatient treatment, but offer intensive outpatient services as well.

Psychiatric hospitals frequently offer AODA treatment. Some specialize in dual diagnosis programs for individuals with a primary psychiatric diagnosis who also abuse alcohol and other drugs. While most of these programs follow traditional inpatient and intensive outpatient programming, others offer more individualized treatment.

Independent clinicians, including psychiatrists, psychologists, social workers, and substance abuse counselors, can offer outpatient AODA treatment. Some clinicians follow a traditional Twelve-Step treatment approach exclusively, while others offer varying degrees of individualized treatment.

IMPLICATIONS

AODA treatment programs can differ along two dimensions which have important clinical implications. First, treatment can be genuinely *individualized* or it can be *program-driven*. Contemporary research supports treatment matching, with interventions tailored to fit each individual client. However, most treatment programs are program-driven and committed to the assumption that all alcoholics and addicts require the same type of treatment. Rehabilitation professionals must be able to evaluate the extent to which a treatment program is willing and able to offer genuinely individualized treatment. Strategies for evaluating these issues are described later in this chapter.

The second important dimension is *treatment intensity*, which can vary from 28-day or longer inpatient treatment to much less intensive outpatient interventions. Conventional wisdom follows a more is better assumption: the more expensive and intensive treatment is, the more effective it will be. However, objective research does not support the presumed therapeutic superiority of longer term treatment in an inpatient setting (Institute of Medicine, 1990; Miller & Hester, 1986a). The length and intensity of treatment is, of course, dependent on the individual client's condition and situation; for some, intensive and/or longer term treatment may well be necessary for recovery. As a general rule, however, more intensive and expensive treatment is *not* necessarily better treatment. When appropriately matched to client needs, less intensive interventions can be the least expensive and most cost-effective (Heather, 1989; Institute of Medicine, 1990; Marlatt, 1988).

There is some evidence that unnecessarily intensive treatment can be counter-therapeutic. A review of the research by the Institute of Medicine of the National Academy of Sciences (1990) concluded that participation in alcoholism treatment is not without risk of harm. The Institute further cautions that drinking problems can actually be *exacerbated* by treatment programs that ignore individual differences and rely on negative confrontational techniques. They concluded that

> Inasmuch as alcohol treatment can result in harm, a reflexive "yes" to the question "Is treatment necessary?" may not only result in the wasteful use of treatment resources (through the delivery of unnecessary or ineffective treatment) but may actually lead to injury, albeit unintentioned. Treatment is therefore not to be taken lightly. (p. 156)

Substance abuse may reflect ecological problems with complex linkages to environmental cues, family dynamics, and social support systems (Blane & Leonard, 1987; Childress, McLellan, & O'Brien, 1986; Moos, Fenn, Billings, & Moos, 1989; Steinglass, 1987). When inpatient treatment is provided in an institutional environment far removed from the realities of clients' lives, they may not be adequately prepared to deal with the real world pressures that await them upon return from treatment; eventual relapse is almost certain. In many cases, the most effective treatment is specifically designed to take advantage of an outpatient setting, using an experiential approach that helps clients learn and practice coping skills at home and work (Gossop, 1989; Institute of Medicine, 1990; Marlatt & Gordon, 1985; Monti, Abrams, Kadden, & Conney, 1989).

Research clearly does not support the notion that more treatment is better treatment. Overtreating a problem with unnecessarily intensive treatment might even harm the client. Case managers are not necessarily acting in the best interest of their clients by reflexively advocating the most intensive treatment available. Effective case management focuses on helping the client gain access to individualized treatment at the appropriate level of intensity–neither too little *nor* too much (Heather, 1989; Institute of Medicine, 1990; Marlatt, 1988).

Rehabilitation professionals can best serve their clients by developing a referral network of AODA treatment programs that can provide assessments and treatment. The next section describes the steps rehabilitation professionals can take to arrange objective assessments and refer their clients to the most appropriate AODA treatment. It includes specific questions intended to help rehabilitation professionals select providers best able to serve the needs of their clients.

ARRANGING OBJECTIVE ASSESSMENTS

The assessment is fundamental to individualized treatment. An objective assessment is based solely on client needs and is free of program biases.

The most common bias is assessor conflict of interest. The clinician performing the assessment should not have any sort of vested interest in promoting one type of treatment over another. The assessor should not stand to gain from recommending inpatient treatment over outpatient, or one program over another. The sole criterion should be the best interest of the client. There is evidence that assessors affiliated with treatment programs tend to recommend the treatment offered by their own facilities (Hansen & Emrick, 1983). Since many inpatient programs were explicitly designed to increase hospital admissions, care most be taken to ensure that assessors are not under pressure to fill empty beds by prescribing unnecessary inpatient treatment.

Individualized treatment requires a comprehensive, multidimensional assessment. It should address (in a meaningful way): (a) alcohol and drug use, (b) problems in other life areas that are caused by AODA, and (c) problems in other life areas that contribute to AODA. The following questions are guidelines to assist in selecting assessors.

The rehabilitation professional should ask "What specific areas are assessed, how, and by whom?" It is critically important to determine *how* each area is assessed. Are important areas assessed by a single open-ended question during an unstructured interview or with formal assessment procedures? Are the assessment procedures standardized and validated or does the assessor rely upon unvalidated questionnaires?

It is likewise important to know the qualifications of the person performing the assessment. Does the assessor have the specialized training needed to assess problems in other life areas such as marital problems, neuropsychological status, sexual dysfunction, and parent-child problems? A substance abuse counselor with a bachelor's degree or less is not likely to have the clinical skills necessary to assess each of these areas in a meaningful way.

Rehabilitation professionals should be wary of narrow drug-centered assessments which assume that substance abuse is always the primary problem. A functional AODA assessment will attempt to identify reciprocal relationships among AODA and other life problems rather than assuming that problems in other life areas are always the result of substance abuse, never the cause.

An assessment should be *differentiating* rather than categorizing. It should ask "How is this person *different* from all others?" instead of trying to reduce a heterogeneous group of people into diagnostic categories. This contrasts with an assessment that assumes that substance abusers are a homogeneous group, with predictable traits, uniform symptomatology, and known progression.

The assessment should provide specific treatment recommendations with explicit goals. It should answer the question "What *specific activities* are being prescribed, and how do those activities address *specific goals*?" The assessment should demonstrate how the recommended treatment activities are functionally related to client goals, avoiding vague global treatment recommendations such as 21-day inpatient alcoholism treatment or six weeks of outpatient treatment. If the assessor assumes that treatment goals and activities are implicit and invariable then the assessment is unlikely to contribute to the developing of a genuinely individualized treatment plan.

The assessment should clearly specify how the treatment recommendations are *matched* to the client. It should explicitly point out the links between the situation and characteristics of the individual client and the specific treatment recommendations. There should be a clear statement of the logical relationship between the assessment results and the treatment recommendations, showing how specific problems or deficits will be addressed by specific therapeutic strategies. A functional assessment will answer the question "Why are you recommending treatment X for individual Y?" rather than assuming that the diagnostic label dictates the treatment.

An assessment meeting the criteria described above should provide detailed and specific information about the client's individual situation, needs, and goals. In order to match the client to the most appropriate treatment, the rehabilitation professional will need to evaluate the services provided by treatment programs.

EVALUATING SERVICES

It is essential that the referring professional directly assess the attitudes of the clinicians. Some treatment programs use marketing staff, sometimes termed "community relations specialists," to promote their services. The picture provided by marketers and administrators might be quite different from that obtained from direct contact with clinicians. When evaluating the services provided by a treatment program, it is critical to talk directly with the clinicians, not only with administrators and marketers.

In order to provide individualized treatment, rehabilitation professionals should select providers who are open to a wide variety of treatment approaches and procedures, but selective in using procedures that have been empirically tested. The following guidelines will be helpful in assessing clinician attitudes: Do the staff evidence flexibility or inflexibility in their treatment approach? Are they dogmatic in their treatment assumptions or are they open to empirically-tested alternatives. Do they reflexively reject procedures that are not part of their established protocol? Is a full range of treatment options available, with procedures tailored to fit the individual?

Are staff concerned with the research evidence supporting approaches and procedures or do they select their procedures solely on the basis of adherence to an ideology? Are they knowledgeable about recent research on controversial topics? Do they acknowledge the research evidence contradicting the homogeneity and one best way assumptions, or do they ignore or deny research evidence that does not support their preferred approach?

How are clients assessed? Does the program use a binary diagnosis (alcoholic/not alcoholic) or an individual and multidimensional assessment? Who does the assessment? Is there a potential for conflict of interest over a wish to fill empty beds?

Is the assessment information used to differentially prescribe specific treatment procedures? To what extent is the treatment protocol individualized? To what extent are all patients expected to conform to a core treatment?

What proportion of clients are referred to Twelve-Step groups? If treatment is based on Twelve-Steps participation, how do clinicians deal with clients who refuse to follow Twelve-Step groups or drop out of the group? What alternative treatment models are offered for persons who do not fit that approach?

What happens when a client does not concur with treatment recommendations? Are theoretical constructs such as denial and lack of motivation used to rationalize treatment failures or does the program develop treatment alternatives?

It is important to assess the clinical competence of the clinicians who will be doing the actual counseling. Most treatment programs have staff with master's, medical, and doctoral degrees but their involvement in actual face-to-face counseling may be minimal. Determine who does the day-to-day counseling, and their credentials. Is most of the actual counseling done by paraprofessional substance abuse counselors without a graduate degree? How many hours per week do patients have fact-to-face contact with master's or doctoral level clinicians? Do physician or psychologist supervisors participate in clinical teams and monitor counselors' clinical skills?

Many substance abusers have few problems early in treatment but relapse weeks or months after treatment is completed. A quality program will have specific procedures in place for relapse prevention. Do the clients learn and practice specific skills for long term maintenance and relapse prevention? If so, what procedures are used? What steps are taken to promote carryover to the real world? A program that assumes that AA is the sole mechanism for relapse prevention incurs the risk that many individuals may drop out of Twelve-Step groups and could be more effective if it also provided alternative relapse prevention strategies.

Rehabilitation professionals can learn much about a treatment program by exploring attitudes towards accountability. Are staff willing to discuss relapse and recidivism rates? How many people go through multiple cycles of treatment? What is the definition of success? Is it based on objective or subjective criteria? How is the information collected? Does the program evaluate its effectiveness through follow-up survey? Are follow-up surveys biased towards favorable results by subtly pressuring former patients to give positive reports of their status? When are clients followed up? Short-term (less than one year after treatment) success rates are often high. What are the results one and two years after treatment?

Is there evidence of selection bias in reporting effectiveness of treatment? Are reported success rates based on *all* persons admitted to treatment, or only those who successfully completed the full regimen? Are persons who refused to comply with treatment and those who dropped out included? How many clients cannot be located at follow-up? Are they included in follow-up statistics? Is the program evaluation based on all clients who entered the program or a small, selected subgroup?

Is client confidentiality used as an excuse to evade accountability? Program effectiveness data can be shared without violating confidentiality. Programs that are reluctant to do so might be revealing their unwillingness to be held accountable for the quality of their services.

Compliance is more likely when clients actively participate in formulation of treatment goals and the intervention is appropriately matched to client (Miller & Hester, 1986b). There is evidence that denial and resistance are much less likely if clients perceive that they are *involved* in treatment decisions, rather than being told what they must do by clinicians (Miller, 1989). The treatment program's attitude toward their clients offers key insights into the extent of client involvement in treatment decisions. Are clients treated as active participants in treatment or passive recipients? Do the staff take a condescending attitude towards their clients? How do they refer to their clients? Do they appear to communicate with their clients in a parent-child or an adult-adult mode? Does the program allow and encourage active case management and open communication with referring counselors and case managers? Is there an attitude that reflects an unwillingness to coordinate services with other professionals who are seeing the client?

Many treatment programs demand that clients accept the alcoholic or addict self-label. However, research has now shown a relationship between acceptance of these self-labels and treatment outcome (Miller, 1989). Nevertheless, many programs rigidly insist that clients accept the self-label, which may provoke resistance and denial.

A problem-solving approach, which focuses on the acquisition of coping skills rather than self-labeling, is much less likely to provoke resistance and more likely to promote adherence to treatment. Rehabilitation professionals should be wary of programs that seem more committed to labeling than to problem solving.

Another valuable criterion for evaluating services is resource allocation. The rehabilitation professional should attempt to estimate the extent to which resources are devoted to clinical activities rather than overhead. Does the program appear to have high overhead expenses, e.g., for expansive grounds, extravagant furnishings, and extensive advertising? While these concerns might seem trivial, unnecessary overhead expenses divert funds from the clinical services, which are far more important to clients' recovery. How much does the service cost? How does that compare to other programs?

Rehabilitation professionals are encouraged to evaluate services assertively, asking direct questions and eliciting feedback from treatment providers. The providers' response to these questions can offer important insights into their willingness to work cooperatively with other professionals. If a provider reacts with an adversarial or defensive posture, that should be a major concern. Confident and competent providers should not be threatened by challenging questions; to the contrary, they should welcome the opportunity to broaden their own perspective by listening to divergent viewpoints. If they react in a hostile or defensive manner, that suggests that they may be primarily concerned with defending their approach rather than allowing their program to evolve and expand to offer the types of treatment an individual client needs. Genuinely individualized treatment is client-centered, and not dedicated to promoting a particular model or approach to treatment.

APPROPRIATE TREATMENT INTENSITY

The previous sections provide guidelines for developing a network of assessment and treatment resources dedicated to providing objective assessments and individualized treatment. The next concern is to ensure that clients receive treatment at an appropriate level of intensity.

As noted previously, more treatment is not necessarily better treatment. Provision of an unnecessarily intensive level of treatment does not promise a superior outcome and might even be counter-therapeutic. However, treatment at an inadequate level of intensity is also unlikely to meet the client's needs. In the simplest terms, the goal is to provide what the client needs but no more. The principle of Least Intensive Appropriate Intervention is a useful guideline for achieving this goal.

This principle of Least Intensive Appropriate Intervention ranks along a continuum of intensity, from minimal interventions such as one or two sessions of feedback and advice, up to inpatient treatment in a hospital (Figure 1). Based on the results of the assessment, the client is referred to the least intensive level of treatment likely to meet his or her needs and produce a positive treatment outcome.

FIGURE 1. Least Intensive Appropriate Intervention

1. Feedback and advice
2. Self-help group
3. Self-help group with minimal counseling
4. Non-intensive counseling
5. Intensive outpatient treatment
6. Outpatient detoxification followed by intensive outpatient treatment
7. Inpatient detoxification (3 to 5 days) followed by intensive outpatient treatment
8. Intensive outpatient treatment with "half-way house" residential support
9. Intensive outpatient treatment with "half-way house" residential support, preceded by in- or outpatient detoxification as indicated
10. Inpatient treatment

This model encourages case managers and treatment providers to conceptualize intervention in terms of *the services the client needs* instead of the services the provider offers. Clients should remain in the more intensive levels of treatment *only* until they are able to move to a less intensive level. If a client fails to make progress at a less intensive level of treatment, a reassessment is indicated to determine whether referral to a more intensive level is necessary. Treatment algorithms such as the *Cleveland Criteria* (Hoffmann, Halikas, & Mee-Lee, 1987) provide objective guidelines for matching client needs and level of intensity, as well as criteria for transfer and discharge.

WHEN APPROPRIATE SERVICES ARE NOT AVAILABLE

In some communities, rehabilitation professionals may not be able to obtain comprehensive and objective assessments or individualized treatment that offers multiple options tailored to the individual. The final section of this chapter will describe alternative strategies a rehabilitation program can consider when appropriate services are either unavailable or inaccessible.

RESOURCE DEVELOPMENT

Securing a Commitment. Once appropriate treatment providers have been identified, rehabilitation professionals will need to assess whether they are willing and able to accommodate the needs of persons with disabilities. Treatment programs may or may not be responsive, depending on individual situational factors such as the program's for-profit or non-profit status, the local supply and demand for AODA treatment, the availability of funds, and reimbursement arrangements.

Most substance abuse treatment programs operate in a competitive environment, with many providers actively seeking opportunities to increase referrals to their programs. Some might be receptive to developing specialty services tailored to accommodating the needs of persons with disabilities. In areas where the demand for AODA services exceeds or matches supply, however, providers may be less interested in developing new programs.

In any case, treatment programs will need some assurance that specialized services for persons with disabilities will be utilized.

They will be reluctant to invest in adaptive equipment or specialized staff training if they fear that the demand for the services is insufficient to generate the revenue necessary to sustain a program. This can create problems when treatment programs need a reliable referral flow but a rehabilitation program is unwilling or unable to commit to a specific referral volume. Health insurers and business coalitions have addressed similar health care problems through the use of a purchaser consortium and preferred provider agreements. Rehabilitation programs might consider adopting a similar strategy.

A rehabilitation consortium may be formed by a group of programs which wish to promote the development of specialized substance abuse programs. While an individual rehabilitation program may not produce the number of referrals needed to maintain a substance abuse program, a consortium usually is able to more accurately project a potential referral volume. The consortium distributes a request for proposals to substance abuse programs, indicating their need for quality programs to serve persons with disabilities. The larger potential referral flow from the consortium could help substance abuse treatment programs recognize the need for specialized services and provide the necessary incentive for program development.

Implementation. After securing a commitment to services for persons with dual disabilities, rehabilitation professionals and advocacy groups can work with treatment programs to provide the consultation and training necessary to develop and implement a dual disability program. Since many substance abuse professionals are specialists with somewhat narrow training, they are not likely to be aware of important disability issues. Some might have unfounded or exaggerated concerns about the needs of persons with disabilities and their program's ability to meet those needs. Concerns about physical accessibility and accommodation may be addressed through consultation and training. There will also be more complicated and sensitive issues that will require ongoing dialog and the development of close working relationships.

Accessibility and Accommodation. In most cases, physical accessibility should not be a major obstacle. Licensure or accreditation requirements for substance abuse treatment programs typically require that physical barriers be minimized. When additional or specialized accommodation is required, rehabilitation programs can offer the same type of consultation and training that they would provide to an employer who wishes to improve workplace accessibility.

Substance abuse treatment programs will need education and advice about adaptive equipment and communication alternatives. Most will be aware of common adaptations such as interpreters and telecommunication devices for persons with hearing impairments, and braille materials. However, they are unlikely to know who provides these services or how they are arranged. Rehabilitation professionals can assist by offering training and advice and introducing treatment programs to the agencies that provide adaptive services.

Some treatment programs will have concerns about nursing requirements for clients with physical disabilities. In many cases, these problems are exaggerated and stem more from a lack of information than unwillingness or inability to accommodate. Treatment programs will benefit from consultation or in-service training that addresses these concerns.

Potential Problem Areas. Medication management is one area which will require close coordination between the substance abuse and rehabilitation sectors. Traditionally, substance abuse treatment programs and self-help groups have discouraged the use of *any* psychoactive drugs by persons in treatment. This has created conflicts when drugs are prescribed by a physician for a medical or psychiatric condition. It is *not* the policy of organized self-help groups such as Alcoholics Anonymous to countermand legitimate medical advice. However, individual members, who may exert considerable influence over others, particularly novices, have been known to do so. There are anecdotal reports of well-intentioned but misinformed group members attempting to dissuade others from using prescribed antidepressant, antipsychotic, or anticonvulsant drugs on the grounds that those drugs interfere with recovery.

The medication problem is an example of a potentially serious conflict that can be easily resolved through dialogue with treatment and self-help groups. Rehabilitation physicians and nurses could provide a valuable service to the substance abuse community through presentations or in-service training, explaining the medical needs of persons with certain disabilities, providing accurate information about the addiction potential of prescribed drugs, and showing how properly managed medication will not necessarily trigger relapse or otherwise hinder recovery.

Sick role issues pose another potential conflict. Many rehabilitation professionals and persons with disabilities believe that excessive identification with the sick role may impede rehabilitation (Krantz, Grunberg, & Baum, 1985). A substance abuse treatment program, on the other hand, may encourage self-labeling and identification as a person who suffers from a disease. Individuals participating in concurrent rehabilitation and substance abuse treatment may receive conflicting messages unless each sector is aware of what the other is doing and coordinating their approaches to the sick role.

As rehabilitation professionals, advocacy groups, and substance abuse treatment programs form relationships, disagreements and conflicts are inevitable. There are four general strategies that can minimize and resolve problems around disability issues. The first is *dialogue*; it is critically important that rehabilitation professionals, advocacy groups, and substance abuse professionals talk with each other. Remote, impersonal referral relationships, with intermittent telephone contact between referral and treatment professionals, will almost certainly lead to misunderstandings and conflicts. Turf problems between disability groups and substance abuse self-help groups are another source of conflict that can be managed through dialogue and personal contact. *Cooperation*, through activities such as mutual consultation and shared in-services, and *coordination*, to ensure each sector knows what the other is doing, will help forge facilitative working relationships. Finally, when all sectors are working toward *mutual goals* using *compatible procedures*, the result will be quality, coordinated services that address the needs of the person with a dual disability.

DEVELOPING A PROGRAM

If quality individualized treatment is not available, or if treatment programs are unwilling or unable to provide services to persons with disabilities, rehabilitation programs should consider developing their own programs. There may, in fact, be several advantages to this option. Creation of an AODA program within a rehabilitation program could facilitate quality assurance and coordination of rehabilitation and AODA services. Housing both programs within the same physical plant would avoid accessibility problems and the expense of duplicating adaptive equipment, and allow easy access to required nursing or medical services.

Depending on needs and resources, services could be provided at any of several levels. Several rehabilitation centers have established comprehensive substance abuse treatment programs within their centers. This would require a core staff of trained counselors, appropriate clinical supervision, and in most cases licensing and/or accreditation. While the investment of effort and resources could be substantial, it is a viable alternative for larger programs with a high incidence of AODA problems among their clients. Development and implementation of this level of programming would require assistance from a consultant experienced in AODA program development. In most states, the agency responsible for licensing AODA programs will offer free or low cost consultation.

Another option is to offer lower intensity AODA services within the rehabilitation program and to refer only those clients who need more intensive services to AODA programs. Some Employee Assistance Programs follow a similar model, offering problem assessment, short-term counseling when indicated, and referral to other providers when more intensive services are needed. Most rehabilitation programs would be able to provide the first four levels of service on the continuum of Least Intensive Appropriate Interventions (feedback and advice, referral to a self-help group, referral to self-help with minimal counseling, and nonintensive counseling) without major investment in new staff or resources. Experienced and credentialed staff members should be able to learn the skills necessary through relatively brief but intensive in-service training.

Rehabilitation programs should also consider informal joint ventures with public mental health agencies and with social workers, psychologists, and other helping professionals in private practice. Most rehabilitation programs have established working relationships with outside professionals who are known to provide quality services. With intensive training, experienced and credentialed professionals with a sound background of clinical skills could develop the additional skills needed to provide more intensive AODA services with a moderate investment of time and funds. The cost of providing intensive training can be made more manageable if a number of agencies and human service professionals collaborate by sharing the cost.

SUMMARY

Rehabilitation professionals play a key role in helping their clients gain access to an appropriate level of individualized substance abuse treatment services. Community treatment resources must be carefully screened to identify those willing and able to provide objective assessments and client-centered services. The development of close working relationships between rehabilitation professionals and treatment providers will help maintain communication and cooperative case management. If appropriate services are not available, rehabilitation programs should consider developing alternative programs to expand the range of treatment options available to persons with disabilities and help them gain access to the type of services most likely to assist in resolving substance abuse problems.

REFERENCES

Blane, H.T., & Leonard, K.E. (1987). *Psychological theories of drinking and alcoholism.* New York: Guilford.

Childress, A., McLellan, A., & O'Brien, C. (1986). Abstinent opiate abusers exhibit conditioned craving, conditioned withdrawal and reductions in both through extinction. *British Journal of Addiction, 81,* 655-660.

Gossop, M. (Ed.). (1989). *Relapse and addictive behavior.* New York: Tavistock-Routledge.

Hansen, J., & Emrick, C. (1983). Whom are we calling "alcoholic"? *Bulletin of the Society of Psychologists in Addictive Behaviors, 2,* 164-178.

Heather, N. (1989). Brief intervention strategies. In R.K. Hester & W.R. Miller (Eds.), *Handbook of alcoholism treatment approaches: Effective alternatives* (pp. 67-80). New York: Pergamon.

Hoffmann, N., Halikas, J., & Mee-Lee, D. (1987). *The Cleveland admission, discharge, and transfer criteria.* Cleveland, Ohio: The Greater Cleveland Hospital Association.

Institute of Medicine. (1990). *Broadening the base of treatment for alcohol problems*. Washington, DC: National Academy Press.

Krantz, D., Grunberg, N., & Baum, A. (1985). Health psychology. *Annual Review of Psychology, 36*, 349-383.

Marlatt, G.A. (1988). Matching clients to treatment: Treatment models and stages of change. In D.M. Donovan & G.A. Marlatt (Eds.), *Assessment of addictive behaviors* (pp. 474-483). New York: Guilford.

Marlatt, G.A., & Gordon, J.R. (1985). *Relapse prevention*. New York: Guilford.

Miller, W.R. (1989). Increasing motivation for change. In R.K.Hester & W.R. Miller (Eds.), *Handbook of alcoholism treatment approaches: Effective alternatives* (pp. 67-80). New York: Pergamon.

Miller, W.R., & Hester, R.K. (1986a). Inpatient alcoholism treatment: Who benefits? *American Psychologist, 41*, 794-805.

Miller, W.R., & Hester, R.K. (1986b). Matching problem drinkers with optimal treatments. In W.R. Miller & N. Heather (Eds.), *Treating addictive behaviors: Processes of change* (pp. 175-204). New York: Plenum.

Monti, P., Abrams, D., Kadden, R., & Cooney, N. (1989). *Treating alcohol dependence*. New York: Guilford.

Moos, R., Fenn, C., Billings, A., & Moos, B. (1989). Assessing life stressors and social resources: Applications to alcoholic patients. *Journal of Substance Abuse, 1*, 135-152.

Steinglass, P. (1987). *The alcoholic family*. New York: Basic Books.

PART IV:
SUMMARY

Chapter 16

Issues and Controversies in Chemical Dependence Services for Persons with Physical Disabilities

Deborah Kiley, PhD
Michael Brandt, PhD

Specific prevention, assessment and treatment issues emerge from topics addressed by contributors to this text which are unique to persons with physical disabilities. For example, a thorough understanding of indications for prescription medication is required, as well as criteria for prescription misuse, in order to accurately assess chemical dependence by persons who rely on medication to manage medical aspects of their disability. Other issues are related to accessibility of treatment services, the need for adaptive equipment, and program adaptability for persons with special physical and communication needs. Substance abuse treatment programs may need to modify their facilities and services in order to provide treatment to persons with physical disabilities. The complex nature of this dual diagnosis necessitates the combined efforts of professionals in various disciplines, including chemical dependence, rehabilitation, education and public policy. An integrated, professional perspective must include an understanding that the patient, family, and community are partners in developing comprehensive rehabilitation programming.

Substance abuse must be addressed early in comprehensive rehabilitation since substance use may impede the rehabilitation process. Addressing substance use requires a thorough evaluation, complete medical and psychological assessment, and the implementation of effective rehabilitation treatment approaches. A holistic approach to rehabilitation, including the assessment of substance use and abuse, is necessary for providing cost-effective, thorough, and effective rehabilitation services. This approach must be fostered by professionals who can deliver rehabilitative services, develop public policy, administer facility procedures, train interdisciplinary staff, plan programs, and deliver services. Treatment which is cost effective requires the integration of chemical dependence assessment, prevention and treatment services within existing rehabilitation programming.

This chapter reviews and integrates the principal issues raised by authors of earlier chapters regarding substance abuse and physical disability. These issues include: (1) the need for specialized services, (2) medical aspects of substance abuse and physical disability, (3) substance abuse assessment strategies, (4) substance abuse treatment approaches, (5) development of integrated programs, (6) provision of specialized staff training and education materials, and (7) financial reimbursement for chemical dependence services.

THE NEED FOR SPECIALIZED SERVICES

A report from the National Institute on Alcohol Abuse and Alcoholism on the planning of treatment services discusses the needs of special populations (McGough & Hindman, 1986). The planning manual has two important criteria for defining special populations: (1) the group must be identified by research as underserved in current treatment programs, and (2) clinical experience and research must demonstrate the necessity for subgroup-specific interventions. The report identifies eight major groups that meet these criteria, including individuals with physical disabilities. This group includes persons with traumatic spinal cord injuries (SCI), traumatic brain injuries (TBI) and individuals with other physical disabilities.

The preceding chapters contain information pertaining to the design of assessment, treatment, and training programs for this special, underserved population. Virtually every author in this book agrees about the need for a multidisciplinary effort. The team of professionals from disciplines who work together should assume responsibility for the special needs of persons with physical disabilities resulting from alcohol and other drugs. Unfortunately, this kind of interdisciplinary endeavor is often lacking and is one of the greatest challenges facing the pioneers in this developing area of rehabilitation. A team approach that provides an interdisciplinary framework in which rehabilitation and chemical dependence professionals can address issues related to substance abuse and physical disability is imperative since substance abuse is so pervasive and affects many facets of individuals' lives.

The need for an interdisciplinary model is highlighted in Kenny Gorman's chapter which describes his experiential account of chemical dependence. One of the most striking issues identified by Gorman is the frequent neglect of patients' pre-injury substance use by rehabilitation professionals. Gorman recalls how his pre-injury substance abuse history was ignored to the extent that he was served "spirits" while in the hospital, and encouraged to drink alcohol in an attempt to wean him from pain medications. He began to use alcohol, marijuana, cocaine, and heroin after discharge from the rehabilitation hospital and reestablished his addiction. Gorman's autobiographical sketch points to several issues for professionals in rehabilitation and chemical dependency: (1) the need for substance abuse professionals to take into account the medical aspects of patients' disabilities, (2) the need for adequate assessment of pre-injury substance use, (3) the importance of early identification of substance abuse problems, (4) the need to coordinate care and enhance communication between physicians, nurses, mental health workers, family members, and other social support systems in the treatment of addiction, and (5) the role of follow-up treatment for both physical disability and chemical dependency. These issues and others are discussed in the following sections.

MEDICAL ASPECTS OF SUBSTANCE ABUSE AND PHYSICAL DISABILITY

Gary Yarkony outlines the process of rehabilitation for persons with traumatic spinal cord injuries, brain injuries, and amputations. He focuses on the medical complications related to rehabilitation outcome which may be affected by post-injury substance abuse. Some medical complications due to substance abuse may result in increased dependency on care providers, a reduction in self-image, and an increase in social isolation. Alcohol or other drug abuse may result in the exacerbation of conditions such as urinary tract infections and pressure sores. Furthermore, the interaction between prescription medications and illicit substances can interfere with the rehabilitation process. Yarkony's discussion makes it clear that comprehensive assessment of alcohol and other drug use is essential, and can help minimize medical complications and enhance rehabilitation planning.

The use of prescription medications by persons with physical disabilities often prohibits the use of alcohol, and requires continued monitoring for side effects. Diazepam (Valium), a short-acting benzodiazepine, is one drug that is commonly prescribed to reduce spasticity, particularly among persons with SCI. The interaction of diazepam and other substances, such as alcohol, is an example of a prescription medication which can produce a profoundly depressing and sometimes fatal effect. Tolerance to the prescribed dose may occur, thus predisposing persons to illicit substance use as adjunctive therapy. Schnoll and Shade-Zeldow emphasize this issue and recognize the need for adequately prescribed dosages, the advantages and disadvantages of narcotic and sedative-hypnotic use, and the need for carefully monitored prescription medication use.

A related controversy is the appropriateness of prescription medications to manage medical complications. Schaschl categorizes prescription medications as being essential or nonessential and disapproves of the use of nonessential, convenience drugs such as mood-altering prescription medications to manage long-term, often chronic conditions such as pain and spasticity. For example, she views antiseizure medication as being essential for the treatment of chronic seizure disorders while questioning the use of sedative-hypnotics and narcotic analgesics. However, Schnoll distinguishes between prescription medication use and misuse, and between dependence and addiction. His view of prescription medication allows for its use as long as it is prescribed and monitored properly. The use of prescription medication remains controversial among rehabilitation professionals and is an issue which consumers, clinicians and researchers must continue to discuss. This issue may best be addressed by utilizing a treatment tailoring approach which is specific to each individual.

SUBSTANCE ABUSE ASSESSMENT STRATEGIES

Traditional assessment of chemical dependence is insufficient to provide the type of comprehensive evaluation of substance use which is needed to make appropriate treatment referrals for persons with physical disabilities. These traditional assessment and diagnostic procedures focus primarily on chemical dependence issues and provide a dichotomous categorization of patients as being either chemically dependent or not chemically dependent. This assessment overlooks the needs of persons who are at risk for chemical dependence and who could benefit from prevention services rather than treatment. For example, the reduced frustration tolerance and impulsivity that often accompanies traumatic brain injury may place persons with a pre-injury alcohol use history at risk for post-injury alcohol abuse. The use of alcohol may impair the effectiveness of rehabilitation and place persons at risk for serious medical complications.

During acute rehabilitation, persons with acquired disabilities are typically provided a rehabilitation treatment plan which is based on medical and psychosocial assessments. For persons with congenital disabilities, medical and psychosocial needs are assessed throughout the life span to provide rehabilitation services and enhance independent functioning. The level of functional independence is enhanced by identifying individuals' strengths and attempting to ameliorate their limitations. Activities of daily living, such as eating, bathing, dressing and mobility, are assessed to determine the current level of functional independence. In addition to these kinds of functional assessments, a comprehensive assessment of alcohol and other drug use will provide information about illicit and prescribed drug use which may interfere with rehabilitation and result in chemical dependence. Cognitive impairment resulting from chemical use may impede learning activities of daily living and developing effective psychosocial coping skills.

An individualized assessment that documents physical, sensory and cognitive limitations will provide the information necessary to make an appropriate referral to a treatment program. Some disabilities may predispose individuals to specific kinds of treatment. The severity of disability may dictate the types of treatment that are appropriate for a particular individual. The level of caregiver assistance required by an individual may determine which treatment options are appropriate and likely to result in favorable treatment outcomes. For example, the treatment of chemical dependence among persons with TBI may be planned differently than for persons with SCI because of cognitive limitations and level of language skills. Rehabilitation professionals can assure that limitations resulting from environmental restrictions are incorporated in treatment planning, too.

Assessment protocols must also take into account interactions between prescribed medications, alcohol, and other drugs. A multidimensional assessment procedure that examines the frequency, intensity and duration of an individuals' drinking behavior in the context of their medical care and social environment would be valuable in making rehabilitation and chemical dependence treatment recommendations. This type of assessment could be developed by members of an interdisciplinary team of professionals, and subject to validation, become a standard assessment instrument for persons with physical disabilities.

SUBSTANCE ABUSE TREATMENT STRATEGIES

Determining when to address substance abuse problems is an unresolved issue. Typically, persons who have sustained traumatic injury must be hospitalized and immediately referred for intensive inpatient and outpatient rehabilitation. It is imperative that acute medical needs are addressed. However, the question remains: How long after a person is medically stable should problems associated with chemical dependency be addressed? Rehabilitation professionals typically address issues such as medical stabilization, proper positioning, range of motion and muscle strengthening, functional independence, discharge planning and adaptive coping skills. How-

ever, alcohol and drug abuse often are not considered primary rehabilitation issues, even when they contribute to injury. One explanation for this practice is that some rehabilitation professionals may
believe that it is not their responsibility. The lack of knowledge
about alcohol and other drugs among professionals also contributes
to these issues not being routinely addressed during rehabilitation.
In addition, some professionals may avoid the issue of alcohol and
other drug abuse because of their own attitudes and the negative
stigma which is associated with chemical dependency. As with
disability-related attitudes, rehabilitation professionals should be
aware of how attitudes about alcohol and other drugs affect their
patient care.

The value of matching patients to appropriate treatment programs is an issue which is emphasized by several authors. Treatment matching consists of identifying salient patient characteristics
and providing individualized treatment in a specific setting, using
the appropriate modality. Important variables to be considered in
treatment matching include social support, marital status, interpersonal style, mood state, locus of control, and level of cognitive
function. Patients with cognitive deficits, such as problems with
memory, concentration, and impulse control, are at greater risk of
relapse than are patients without these deficits. Thomas Budziack
provides an in-depth discussion of treatment matching and practical
techniques which clinicians may use to match patients to treatment
programs. Skinner (1984) has also incorporated many of these variables in his design of a sophisticated treatment matching program;
he provides a psychometrically sound assessment instrument, the
Treatment Goals Inventory (Glasser & Skinner, 1981). While treatment matching is a compelling strategy, there is little outcome data
available on programs that use treatment matching strategies.

Appropriate matching of patients to treatment programs is a first
step toward providing effective treatment for chemical dependence.
In addition, the value of involving families in the assessment and
treatment of chemical dependence is raised by several authors.
Family members can provide collateral information about a patient's use and abuse of alcohol which may allow for early intervention. The inclusion of families in rehabilitation and chemical depen-

dence programming can also enhance the treatment process and effectiveness.

Future research should examine treatment matching factors that are germane to populations with physical disabilities. For example, factors such as communication skills, cognitive function and physical mobility may be salient treatment matching variables. Traditional methods of treating persons with chemical addictions are also poorly researched. It is only through the evaluation of traditional programs and treatment matching strategies that the field will be able to confidently match patients to treatment modalities with a high degree of success. For example, individuals with cognitive impairments or learning disabilities may require adapted programming. Educational lectures and group therapy are two major components of traditional treatment programs, yet both of these approaches may be ineffective for persons with memory deficits, decreased attention span, and problems with concentration and encoding of information. Persons with TBI may require shorter individual and group sessions, more individualized sessions, information presented several times, and simplified written materials. In addition, certain conditions, such as cognitive, visual, or auditory impairment, may require the use of specialized assessment tools and intervention modalities, such as the use of illustrations or tape recordings.

PROGRAM DEVELOPMENT

The accessibility of chemical dependence facilities often determines which treatment programs are utilized by persons with disabilities. Accessibility refers to the architectural and programmatic accommodations which are required by individuals with disabilities in order to participate fully in the treatment program. Architectural accommodations include ramps, wider doorways and accessible bathrooms. Programmatic accommodations include provision of interpreters and TTY devices for persons who are deaf, and braille translations for persons who are blind. Individuals who have cognitive deficits may require other accommodations such as shorter or more structured sessions, lower reading level materials or illustrated materials, and frequent repetition of information. Doot as well as Schaschl and Dennis Straw describe programs that have made programmatic changes to accommodate persons with physical disabilities; Blackerby and Baumgarten (1990) present a treatment program designed to provide holistic rehabilitation services to persons with TBI who were diagnosed as being chemically abusive or dependent. These programs may be used as examples in developing other accessible chemical dependence program accommodations.

TRAINING PROFESSIONALS

Education of rehabilitation professionals in substance abuse and the education of substance abuse treatment professionals in physical disability remain critical issues. Substance abuse prevention, intervention and treatment could be made considerably more available for persons with disabilities through existing rehabilitation services. Due to the inevitable involvement with health care services and rehabilitation professionals, persons with physical disabilities may come in contact with health care providers more frequently than does the general population.

Training, treatment and referral procedures will vary between facilities depending on their patient populations and the availability of chemical dependence treatment services. Suitable training materials for professionals working with this population remain limited. Attitudes held by staff about alcohol and other drugs can undermine the utilization of assessment and treatment resources. It is imperative that rehabilitation professionals receive education which will impact both knowledge and attitudes about alcohol and other drug use among patients. An example of this education is a program developed at the Rehabilitation Institute of Chicago. This facility provides ongoing staff training about alcohol and other drugs so that these issues are addressed systematically by new staff during rehabilitation. Discipline-specific educational materials are being developed which are tailored to various staff roles and types of patient care.

FINANCIAL REIMBURSEMENT

The question of who pays for chemical dependence treatment is often a difficult issue for persons with physical disabilities. Insurance coverage may end just when a referral to a chemical dependence treatment facility becomes appropriate. Blackerby and Baumgarten (1990) identified the lack of adequate funding, including third-party payments, as being responsible for 83% of referrals being ineligible for services. There was agreement between insurance case managers and referring social workers that services were necessary and that the program was greatly needed; however, funding support from patients' insurance was often unavailable. If included as part of the overall rehabilitation program, substance abuse treatment would pose less of a funding problem for patients. Attention to substance abuse issues could be integrated into existing rehabilitation programming, such as disability adjustment and sexuality topics, which would not require a separate chemical dependence treatment program.

Third-party payment is more often available for traditional in-patient and out-patient alcohol and drug abuse treatment. Treatment fees vary depending on whether treatment is available within the rehabilitation setting or arranged through existing chemical dependence treatment programs. However, it is often the case that individuals with physical disabilities are not appropriate for traditional chemical dependence treatment due to behavior problems, cognitive impairments, limited architectural accessibility, and other limitations discussed earlier. Thus, other treatment options must be made available both clinically and financially.

SUMMARY

This chapter has identified the primary issues and controversies regarding substance abuse as they apply to persons with physical disabilities. The first controversy reviewed was the question of specialized assessment and treatment services. This discussion supports the concept of specialized services based on the need for adaptive treatment modalities, accessible facilities and effective prevention strategies. The medical aspects of physical disability and the use of prescription medication pose another controversy. Consequently, the use of prescription medication may be viewed as one aspect of assessment which requires individualized evaluation.

Assessment and treatment of substance abuse should be provided as early as possible in the rehabilitation process. The assessment of substance abuse should take place during the initial evaluation and in routine follow-up evaluations, and should reflect a comprehensive, interdisciplinary effort. Substance abuse treatment may be integrated into existing rehabilitation programs, and patients may be matched to chemical dependence treatment programs considering their special characteristics. Successful program development in which the specific needs of persons with physical disabilities are addressed requires thoughtful adaptation, programmatic flexibility, and architectural accessibility. Interdisciplinary models of staff education in combination with the demonstration of administrative support will enhance the efficacious training of both rehabilitation and chemical dependence professionals. Finally, if substance abuse treatment is integrated into existing rehabilitation programs, the cost for treatment may become part of overall rehabilitation and thereby enhance cost containment.

Substance abuse and physical disability remain important issues for professionals, patients, and family members to address. This chapter, and those preceding it, have merely begun to address the complexities and gravity of these issues. Excellence in patient care demands further exploration, considerable attention, and continued research.

REFERENCES

Blackerby, W.F. & Baumgarten, A. (1990). A model treatment program for the head injured substance abuser: Preliminary findings. *Journal of Head Trauma Rehabilitation, 3*, 47-59.

Glasser, F.B. & Skinner, H.A. (1981). Matching in the real world: A practical approach. In E.A. Gottheil, A.T. McLellan & K.A. Druley (Eds.). *Matching patient needs and treatment methods* (pp 295-324). Springfield, IL: Charles C Thomas.

McGough, D.P. & Hindman, M. (1986). *A guide to planning alcoholism treatment programs*. Rockville, MD: National Institute on Alcohol Abuse and Alcoholism.

Skinner, H.A. (1984). An overview of the core-shell treatment system. In F.B. Glaser, H.M. Annis, H.A. Skinner, S. Pearlman, R.L. Segal, B. Sisson, A.C. Ogborne, E. Bohnen, P. Gazda & T. Zimmerman (Eds.) *A System of Health Care Delivery*, vol. 1. (pp. 17-26). Toronto: Addiction Research Foundation.

Index